# HOSPICE CONCEPTS

## A Guide to Palliative Care in Terminal Illness

## Shirley Ann Smith

**Research Press**
2612 North Mattis Avenue
Champaign, Illinois 61822
www.researchpress.com

DISCLAIMER

> This publication is intended to offer guidelines of care. The information contained in this publication is not meant as a substitute for supervised training, instruction, or accreditation, and the completion or review of the information set forth in this publication does not imply any type of certification or competency. The publisher and the author will not be held liable for or responsible for individual treatments, specific plans of care, patient and family outcomes, or inadvertent errors or omissions in the text. The publisher and the author neither assume nor authorize any person to assume for the publisher and the author any other liability in connection with the sale or use of the information contained in this publication.

Chapter tests appearing in Appendix A may be reproduced for instructional use only. Excerpts may be printed in connection with published reviews in periodicals without express permission. No other part of this book may be reproduced by any means without the written permission of the publisher.

Copies of this book may be ordered from the publisher at the address given on the title page.

Cover design by Publication Services, Inc.

Composition by Jeff Helgesen

Printed by Bang Printing

ISBN 0–87822–453–X

Library of Congress Catalog Number 00–133931

*To my husband, Clair, without whom my life*
*would not be complete, and neither would this book*

# Contents

# Tables

# Foreword

Care for the dying and bereaved in the United States has greatly improved in the past decade, though there are still too many, far too many, patients and families who receive less-than-optimal care. Good care at the end of life is every person's right, not a privilege reserved for the fortunate few. Hospices and other palliative care programs have contributed much to the improvement in end-of-life care, but their proliferation has increased the need for sound professional education. This book makes a significant contribution to such education.

Good hospice and palliative care requires the consistent and compassionate application of sound basic principles. Our fascination with the latest variants of technology and pharmacology too often leads us to forget what matters most in caring for the dying and the bereaved: respect for both patient and family members, good symptom control, reliance on the team approach, and emphasis on the quality of the life that is left. This book is a useful guide, and a timely reminder, of the practical principles that are the essential foundation to good hospice and palliative care.

Shirley Smith brings to this book a wealth of professional experience, coupled with personal empathy and understanding. As a nurse and former hospice director, an educator and a consultant to hospices, she understands the challenges of providing good patient care in diverse environments. She knows firsthand the type of information and education needed by all members of the multiprofessional teams working with the dying and the bereaved. This book not only offers extensive information about a variety of patient care issues encountered daily in hospice and palliative care, it also captures the values and the spirit that set such care apart, and to which all of us, as caregivers at the end of life, should aspire.

MICHAL GALAZKA
EXECUTIVE DIRECTOR
HOSPICE EDUCATION INSTITUTE
ESSEX, CONNECTICUT

# Preface

This hospice guide was written to fill a void. Although there are many excellent texts available on hospice care, none gives a succinct, yet comprehensive, overview. The works of authors such as Cicely Saunders, Derek Doyle, Jack Zimmerman, Peter Kaye, Charles Kemp, Robert Enck, and others have become standard references. Edited by Doyle, Hanks, and MacDonald, the *Oxford Textbook of Palliative Medicine*, a definitive text describing the results of several decades of concentrated practice and a considerable body of research, was published in 1993, and the revised second edition appeared in 1998.

What strikes me as we see the proliferation of excellent books on palliative care is that those interested in palliative care are becoming more mature in their knowledge and insights, but those unfamiliar with palliative care are being left out—left out in the sense that a book with lengthy detail on a myriad of hospice topics would not appeal to the uninitiated. Clinicians in general practice or in specialties other than hospice, approaching hospice ideas for the first time, will want information about its basic tenets. For example, we have a plethora of in-depth pain management texts, yet what is needed for pain management in terminally ill patients is a better understanding of basic guidelines for effective use of familiar analgesics.

The original idea for this book germinated as I heard from hospice team members across the country that they began working in hospice without benefit of an orientation program. It seems hard to believe that this could happen, given the level of sophistication that hospice has achieved in the past 25 years. Well-developed orientation programs are available, both from hospice professionals and from commercial medical education firms. There may be various reasons these programs are not more widely used, including the complexity of the texts, the need to provide an instructor, cost of the materials, or cost of staff classroom time.

It became obvious to me that there is a widespread need for an affordable yet inclusive overview of hospice concepts. As an orientation manual, this book can be used for groups or for individual self-study (which may be a practical thing to do if only one or two new employees are joining the staff). Chapter tests and answers for evaluation purposes are included in two appendixes.

Various chapters—for example, on spiritual concerns or communication skills—could be used for staff inservices. The book also can be used by staff as a reference manual, especially the information on pain management, therapeutic interventions for common symptoms, and imminent death. The text applies to all disciplines because hospice team success depends on all team members' understanding the broad concepts and developing the flexibility to be supportive of one another while working toward meeting the needs of patients and families.

While I was in the process of writing this book, I read the report published by the Institute of Medicine entitled *Approaching Death: Improving Care at the End of Life*. This study indicated that despite the impact of hospice programs and palliative medicine, as medical technology continues to advance, many practitioners succumb to the temptation to ignore its limits and instead pursue futile treatments for dying patients. Recommendations focus on identifying and limiting futile treatments, pursuing opportunities to better understand the pathophysiology of physical and emotional symptoms in patients with life-threatening illness, and providing reliable, effective, and humane care at this point in the normal cycle of human life.

Based on the Institute of Medicine's recommendations and those of many other national organizations that are promoting improved end-of-life care, professionals in a variety of settings are showing an increased interest in these issues and looking for guidance as they develop palliative care practices in their facilities. In addition, the Joint Commission on Accreditation of Health Care Organizations (JCAHCO) began several years ago to include requirements that address adequate pain management, spiritual needs, and psychosocial distress. These requirements apply to any health care facility having JCAHCO accreditation: acute care hospitals, major medical centers, nursing homes, and so on.

This movement to improve end-of-life care, regardless of setting, has also stimulated interest in curriculum development on palliative care in medical schools and schools of nursing. Accordingly, as I developed this text, I included goals, objectives, and a content outline for each chapter to accommodate academic settings as well as individuals who might apply for continuing education credits. *Hospice Concepts* is purposefully brief to increase usability, but it presents specific, pertinent information that can be applied to daily practice with therapeutic results.

Others who will benefit from a concise overview are doctors and nurses preparing to take hospice and palliative care certification exams. No single text suffices for this kind of preparation. However, an overview of all the essential components is a good beginning. Depending upon their individual responsibilities as team members, some may not have exposure to all the elements that might be covered on certification board exams. So this text covers everything from hospice philosophy to Medicare regulations, from criteria for determining prognosis to dealing with grief and bereavement.

For further study, I have added a list of references and suggested readings at the end of each chapter. These lists include current major resources; some older references are included when they explain historical perspective or are classics that remain pertinent and valid. Some examples of the latter are the works of Elisabeth Kübler-Ross, Sigmund Freud, Cicely Saunders, Herman Feifel, Earl Grollman, and Colin Murray Parkes.

For the sake of clarity, I would like to comment on some of the terminology used in this book. First is my use of the word *family*. I think we have all come to understand that there is no such thing as a "normal" family, as that idea applies to either structure or function. Each patient will define family differently. I use the word to mean all the significant people who surround and are important to each individual patient. It will also be noted that I make no distinction between the phrases *hospice care* and *palliative care*. For the purpose of this book, I see them as having the same meaning. However, one of the differences between these two types of care is prognosis, or life expectancy. Since hospice began, the limited prognosis of 6 months or less has defined which patients are appropriate for hospice. Because Medicare adheres to this definition, that time span will continue to be a hospice admission criteria unless, or until, Medicare regulations change. Palliative care outside of hospice is broader, without this restriction, but subject to reimbursement difficulties. This text focuses on understanding the needs of the dying and on how best to meet those needs, regardless of the setting or method of payment.

Professionals encountering this material for the first time may perceive the palliative approach described as being very conservative. It is conservative if that means minimizing technology and maximizing the practical and human elements of caring for the patient. If our approaches are primarily technological, we may hide behind this activity while ignoring the real needs of the dying. In addition, experience has demonstrated that a holistic, humane approach optimizes the potential for quality of life.

I use the term *technology* here to mean more than machinery and invasive therapies. It also includes diagnostic studies and medication regimens. As per the National Hospice Organization, no specific therapy is excluded from consideration in palliative care. However, the challenge for all of us is the use of integrity in our decision making. When we recommend a therapy or test, we need to be conscious of our motives and determine that the therapy or test is truly in the patient's best interest, and not just to make us look heroic. In the final analysis, successful palliative care at the end of life is measured by how comfortable patients are and how well their goals and values are addressed.

**REFERENCES**

Doyle, D., Hanks, G. W. C., & MacDonald, N. (Eds.). (1993). *Oxford textbook of palliative medicine*. Oxford, England: Oxford University Press.

Doyle, D., Hanks, G. W. C., & MacDonald, N. (Eds.). (1998). *Oxford textbook of palliative medicine* (2nd ed.). New York: Oxford University Press.

Institute of Medicine. (1997). *Approaching death: Improving care at the end of life*. Washington, DC: National Academy Press.

# Acknowledgments

I would like to offer my sincere appreciation and gratitude to many people who were instrumental in making this book a reality. If I were to list everyone who influenced my love and dedication to the work of hospice, I would have to name all the patients and their families who have taught me what really matters when dealing with a life-threatening illness. I would have to name all of the wonderful hospice team members with whom I worked at the Wilkes-Barre, Pennsylvania, Veterans Administration Medical Center, because we grew together as we provided care, studied the literature, carried on research, and taught others. The list could get very long. Obviously, I must limit remarks here to those special people who played key roles in making this book possible.

My husband, Clair, has always been my biggest fan and my major source of encouragement and support. He has always gone the extra mile to make sure that anything mechanical is operating properly, from my car to my computer printer. Beyond that, he has done whatever was needed to allow me to focus my energies on this project. Sometimes that was cooking and household chores; sometimes it was just being patient or making a pot of coffee.

David Zarambo was that special friend who pushed and bugged me to get moving when my courage waned at the awesome thought of writing a book. He also had a special way with my computer when it did not want to cooperate.

I am very grateful to those experts in hospice care who were willing to review the text for accuracy and comprehensiveness. Kay Korb, certified hospice nurse par excellence, proofed many chapters and contributed many helpful ideas. Dr. Salvatore Scialla, oncologist and palliative care physician, reviewed and offered suggestions on the symptom management and pain chapters. Brian Thomas, hospice administrator, generously offered ideas for improving the chapter on Medicare. The expertise of Maria Andrews, dietitian extraordinaire, enhanced the chapter on nutrition and hydration.

The fastidious proofreading of Evelyn Tomasovic and Mark VanValin greatly improved the readability of the manuscript. Neither of them comes from a health care background, so reviewing this kind of material must have been a tedious task, but they cheerfully used a lot of red ink to improve syntax, punctuation, clarity, and all those good things that are obvious to masters of the English language.

Without the help of Pat McCue and Denise Vonderheid, I would have spent even more hours than I did at the computer keyboard. Both of them not only contributed their computer skills but also offered encouragement and enthusiasm.

Jay Suffren and Irene Miller, professional staff at the Wilkes-Barre VA Medical Center library, were always pleasant and efficient in locating valuable resources.

And last but not least, I am grateful to Ann Wendel at Research Press for recognizing the value of this material and to my editor, Karen Steiner, who know so well how to make a manuscript into a book.

# CHAPTER 1

# Hospice Philosophy, History, and Goals

**PURPOSE**

The purpose of this chapter is to provide an overview of the philosophy of palliative care, a history of the development of the modern hospice movement, and a discussion of how the unique goals of palliative care influence practice.

**OBJECTIVES**

Upon completion of this chapter, the learner will be able to:

1. Discuss the evolution of the hospice movement

2. Outline basic hospice philosophy

3. Articulate the difference between patients receiving acute care and patients receiving hospice care

**CONTENT OUTLINE**

I. Hospice Philosophy and Principles of Care

    A. Definition

    B. Basic principles

    C. Key concepts

II. History of Modern Hospice Development

    A. Early models

    B. St. Christopher's Hospice

    C. Development in the United States

# HOSPICE PHILOSOPHY AND PRINCIPLES OF CARE

## Definition

*Hospice* means "given to hospitality." A medieval term, it refers to a resting place for travelers along pilgrim routes, where the sick, the poor, and those weary from traveling were taken in and received care. In modern-day society, *hospice* means a system of specialized care that provides shelter and comfort for the most difficult of journeys—facing one's own death.

In 1990, with growing public and professional concern about the continuing lack of good pain management, especially in terminal cancer patients, the World Health Organization (WHO) became involved. They published a report called "Cancer Pain Relief and Palliative Care" (WHO, 1990). The report suggests the following definition of palliative care:

> Palliative care is the active total care of patients whose disease is not responsive to curative treatment. Control of pain, of other symptoms, and of psychological, social and spiritual problems, is paramount. The goal of palliative care is achievement of the best quality of life for patients and their families. (p. 11)

All hospice programs have some guiding philosophy and/or definition, which describes what can be done, never what cannot be done. Following is one of the most meaningful:

> Hospice affirms life. Hospice exists to provide support and care for persons in the last phases of incurable disease so that they might live as fully and comfortably as possible. Hospice recognizes dying as a normal process whether or not resulting from disease. Hospice neither hastens nor postpones death. Hospice exists in the belief that, through appropriate care and the promotion of a caring community sensitive to their needs, patients and their families may be free to attain a degree of mental and spiritual preparation

for death that is satisfactory to them. (National Hospice Organization, 1993, p. iii)

The Last Acts Task Force on Palliative Care (1997), funded by the Robert Wood Johnson Foundation, defines palliative care as referring to

> the comprehensive management of the physical, psychological, social, spiritual and existential needs of patients. It is especially suited to the care of people with incurable, progressive illnesses. Palliative care affirms life and regards dying as a natural process that is a profoundly personal experience for the individual and family. The goal of palliative care is to achieve the best possible quality of life through relief of suffering, control of symptoms and restoration of functional capacity while remaining sensitive to personal, cultural and religious values, beliefs and practices. (p. 1)

## Basic Principles

When dying is accepted as a normal process, intensive caring instead of intensive care is a more appropriate approach. This does not mean nothing more can be done. It does mean compassionate expertise is applied to relieve or palliate physical, emotional, spiritual, or social discomfort. Aggressive curative medical treatment often may be inappropriate and result in a prolongation of suffering, minimalization of the quality of life, and neglect of patients' priorities. The coordinated program of palliative and supportive care offered by hospice responds to the needs of dying patients by providing an alternative to aggressive, cure-oriented care. The focus of the plan of care is on quality of life, alleviation of distressing symptoms, and bereavement support.

The hospice philosophy does not condone nor participate in any action intended to hasten or prolong a patient's death. Rather, all aspects of care are intended to bring comfort, to celebrate life, and to optimize the patient's control and autonomy. The patient and family are involved in decision making and are provided with enough information about the disease and the options so an informed choice can be made.

## Key Concepts

Certain key concepts should be reflected in all hospice programs. These ideas were formulated by Dr. Cicely Saunders, founder of St. Christopher's Hospice in England, and continue to be widely accepted as necessary to a successful hospice program. Dr. Saunders taught that holistic or comprehensive care must include counseling and team availability to support the patient and family. She also observed that at the end of life, spiritual and emotional pains can be equal to or greater than physical pains. The National Hospice Organization (NHO), founded in 1978, has played a major role in promulgating these concepts by providing educational activities and resources for hospice management. The same concepts have been reflected in Medicare regulations since the program's inception in 1982. Specifically, these concepts are as follows:

- Comprehensive care with continuity between settings
- Patient and family as unit of care
- Physician supervision
- Interdisciplinary team approach
- Around-the-clock availability
- Utilization of volunteers
- Bereavement counseling
- Symptom management
- Spiritual and psychosocial support
- Staff training and support

# HISTORY OF MODERN HOSPICE DEVELOPMENT

## Early Models

The underlying assumptions of the hospice movement are not new. As early as 1879, the Irish Sisters of Charity opened a facility for the sole purpose of "caring for the sick and incurables." In 1905, they opened St. Joseph's Hospice in London. Calvary Hospital in the Bronx, New York, opened in 1899 to deliver a specialized program of care to those with advanced cancer. Calvary Hospital is an important predecessor to today's hospices and has contributed valuable information on care of the dying. While developing plans for St. Christopher's Hospice, Dr. Cicely Saunders visited Calvary Hospital and discussed its work. In recent years, Calvary Hospital has developed professional training programs geared toward the care of patients with advanced cancer.

## St. Christopher's Hospice

Dr. Cicely Saunders, who was first educated as a nurse and as a social worker, then as a physician, became increasingly concerned about how dying patients were treated, and often neglected, in traditional hospital settings. In the 1950s, as the first full-time medical officer at

St. Joseph's Hospice in London, Dr. Saunders became convinced that pain in dying individuals was unnecessary and determined to correct generally accepted practices of the day. Her ideas led to a whole new system of terminal care.

In 1967, Dr. Saunders established St. Christopher's Hospice in London to relieve suffering by developing methods of care, analyzing knowledge, and carrying out research into the control of the physical, mental, and social distress of chronic and long-term illness. St. Christopher's not only offered good pain management and expert physical care, it developed components not previously seen as part of a care plan: family counseling, grief work, follow-up bereavement care, attention to spiritual care, and individualized attention to patient/family values and belief systems. From the beginning, Dr. Saunders focused on serious research and educational programs to increase the knowledge base for care of the dying. Thus was born the modern hospice movement.

## Development in the United States

### Elisabeth Kübler-Ross

At about the same time in the United States, many significant events occurred. The field of thanatology, the study of the effects of death and dying, began to blossom in the midst of a death-defying society. The pioneer in promoting talk about death was Dr. Elisabeth Kübler-Ross. As a young psychiatrist, she developed an interest in working with dying patients, whose needs were so often ignored. She saw the challenge as helping them die "by trying to help them live, rather than vegetate in an inhumane manner" (1969, p. 21).

Kübler-Ross published *On Death and Dying* in 1969. It was not her first book on this topic, but it is probably the most widely quoted. The subtitle, *What the Dying Have to Teach Doctors, Nurses, Clergy, and Their Own Families*, demonstrates her experience that it need not be a dreaded thing to interact with and bring comfort to a dying person. Rather, she relates that the dying are eager to have someone with whom they can share their feelings, their journey, and their needs. She observed similarities in the patterns, or stages, of emotional adjustment that patients experience and described these patterns as denial, anger, bargaining, depression, and acceptance. (These stages will be discussed further in chapter 6.) She also concluded that patients are aware of the seriousness of their conditions but choose to deal with the situation in their own way.

### Other Thanatologists

During the two decades of the 1960s and 1970s, numerous significant studies and publications increased public awareness of death and dying. Most of the articles and books focused on personal development, but they also emphasized the need for openness with others concerning the dying experience. Dr. Herman Feifel, a psychiatrist at the Veterans Hospital in Los Angeles, published several books on the topic. In *New Meanings of Death,* he addressed the societal and learned cultural aversion to discussing death and dying and the impact of this aversion throughout the life span. He also made the poignant observation that "an impersonal technology alienates us from traditional moorings" and weakens institutional and community supports. The consequences, he said, are "increased loneliness, anxiety, and self-pity" (Feifel, 1977, p. 4).

Others at this time publishing pertinent studies, articles, and books included Dr. Avery Weisman, Jeanne Quint, Robert Kastenbaum, and Edwin Shneidman.

### The First American Hospices

The groundwork for translating the needs of the dying into the reality of providing care began in New Haven, Connecticut. During the late 1960s, in an attempt to define these needs, Florence Wald, former Dean of Nursing at Yale University, began collecting data on the thoughts and feelings of dying patients. She and others interested in developing hospice care attended lectures at Yale University given by Dr. Cicely Saunders. The group decided to develop a hospice care program modeled after St. Christopher's in London. The Connecticut Hospice, originally Hospice, Inc., opened in 1974 as a home care hospice program. Program developers eventually built a 52-bed inpatient unit and education center.

Shortly after the opening of the first American hospice, the Hospice of Marin County opened in San Francisco. Subsequent growth of hospice care in the United States was inevitable. By the end of 1978, there were 59 operational hospice programs; in 1998, there were approximately 3,000 (National Hospice Organization, 1999).

The biggest problem in providing a health care service not historically covered by insurance or by government subsidy has been finding adequate funding sources. Though most hospices still do fundraising to cover the uninsured or for special programs, the number of hospice providers increased greatly when Medicare began coverage for hospice care in 1983. Details of the Medicare Hospice Benefit and concomitant guidelines and requirements will be discussed in chapter 12.

There are many models of hospice care, including freestanding units, scattered beds within a hospital, and home health agency hospices that concentrate on care in the home and contract for inpatient services as needed. The last model is by far the most common. But as early hospice writer Sandol Stoddard (1992) wrote, it is not the architecture or the model that makes hospice. Stoddard says hospice is a philosophy of care that begins with the question "What does this patient need?"

# GOALS OF HOSPICE CARE

## Needs of Dying Patients

The goals in hospice care are predicated on what dying patients have taught us about what matters most to them. While the list will vary with individual priorities, it usually includes the following:

+ To maintain control over their environment

+ To have enduring expert physical care

+ To be assured that they and their families won't be abandoned

+ To achieve peace of mind

The goals of hospice relate directly to meeting those needs. Giving priority to the dying person's right to maintain control over the environment, including plan of care, results in the turning of attention toward the patient's values and priorities instead of someone else's. Traditionally, clinicians have looked to lab values or other diagnostic studies to guide their decision making, usually with little or no input from the patient. One of the goals of palliative care is to involve the patient in decision making to the extent he or she desires. If the patient is incompetent, whether from physical or mental incapacity, decisions should be based on what this particular patient would have wanted.

The goal of enduring expert physical care means applying all the art and science of medicine to alleviate and/or prevent distressing symptoms. This goal encompasses knowledge of the social sciences as well as the medical. In the past, clinicians had not studied the dying process and its accompanying signs and symptoms. From the first days of the modern hospice movement, Dr. Cicely Saunders promoted education and research to foster ways to assess the pathophysiology of dying, as well as knowledge of when an intervention is therapeutic. This body of knowledge continues to grow, with an increase in scholarly papers and research studies.

Just as important as expert medical care is the assurance to patients and families that they will not be abandoned by their health care providers. Most patients prefer to continue with the physician they have come to know and trust over time, even when curative treatment is no longer the goal. Physicians are encouraged to remain as the attending to oversee the palliative plan of care when patients are referred to hospice. If a physician is uncomfortable in this role, transition to another doctor to manage the end-of-life care should be worked out with the patient. Nonabandonment also includes the ongoing presence or availability of all hospice team members as needed. The quality and quantity of attention to terminally ill patients should increase rather than decrease. The mere presence of a caring person who is interested in helping to ease suffering has tremendous therapeutic value for patients and their families.

The goal of achieving peace of mind will be defined differently by every individual. There will even be those who will choose not to have this as a goal. Some dying patients will refuse to deal with unfinished business—personal, social, or spiritual. If that is their choice, hospice team members should not personalize this decision or interpret it as failure. Not every patient dies peacefully.

On the other hand, many patients do work at righting wrongs and mending relationships. For some it is a time and opportunity for healing, even though cure is impossible. In Kübler-Ross's (1975) book *Death: The Final Stage of Growth* she concludes from her experience in working with dying patients that coming to terms with death as a part of human development can be a positive experience of inner growth.

In his book *Dying Well: The Prospect for Growth at the End of Life*, Dr. Ira Byock (1997) states that "when people are relatively comfortable and know that they are not going to be abandoned, they frequently find ways to strengthen bonds with people they love and to create moments of profound meaning in their final passage" (p. xiv). He suggests the dying person can reach "developmental landmarks" such as experiencing love of self and others, completing relationships, accepting the finality of one's life, and achieving a new sense of self despite one's impending demise. Although this growth process may involve personal struggle, even suffering, people can grow in ways that are important to them and their families.

## Contrasting the Goals of Hospice and Acute Curative Care

We have grown so accustomed to relying on technology and intensive care units for the care of seriously ill people that the large majority of Americans die in hospitals. However, many studies now indicate that the mechanical and technical approach to patient care prevalent in hospitals today has no beneficial effect for incurably ill patients. Even the basic philosophy, organization, and work patterns of acute care are frequently at odds with the needs of dying patients. Table 1.1 outlines some of the differences.

Psychiatrist Colin Murray Parkes, well known for his studies on bereavement, states that a busy hospital is not a good place to die

## Table 1.1   Differences between Acute Care and Hospice Care

|  | ACUTE CARE | HOSPICE CARE |
|---|---|---|
| **Objective:** | Quantity of life | Quality of life |
| **Philosophy:** | Curative | Palliative |
| **Goal:** | Control of disease | Control of symptoms |
| **Focus:** | Disease | Person |
| **Death seen as:** | Failure | Inevitable, natural |
| **Treatment depends on:** | Lab values, diagnostic studies | Patient symptoms and goals |
| **Unit of care:** | Patient | Patient, family, significant others |
| **Results measured by:** | Cure rates, improved lab values, discharge to home | Freedom from pain, productive activity, peaceful death |

"because the staff are preoccupied with heroic efforts to save life and the patient who cannot be saved is a failure for all" (1996, p. 152). Elisabeth Kübler-Ross observed that the dying patient in an acute care setting "may cry for rest, peace, and dignity, but he will get infusions, transfusions, a heart machine, or a tracheotomy" (1969, p. 9). Dr. Cicely Saunders (1995) observed that the terminal patient's world gets smaller and smaller and the need to be treated as a living, valued human being gets larger and larger. Dying patients need more attention, not less, and they need to relate to the living. Sandol Stoddard (1992) has written:

> The dying have the right to a great many things that institutions cannot provide. They need life around them, spiritual and emotional comfort and support of every sort. They need "unsanitary" things like a favorite dog lying on the foot of the bed. They need their own clothes, their own pictures, music, food, surroundings that are familiar to them, people they know and love, people they can trust to care about them. (p. 63)

And so, the first goal for those of us who work with dying patients is to provide the setting and philosophy of care that meets patient/family needs. The terminally ill patient needs to be in a setting of his or her choice, where the inevitable progression of a disease is understood and intervention is directed toward quality of survival.

Sensitivity and responsiveness to constantly changing needs are part of this caring environment, and what is important to the patient determines that individual's regimen of care. With increased public awareness of a person's right to refuse futile aggressive treatment and increasing knowledge that hospice care can provide the support that it takes to be able to remain at home, more people are choosing this option.

## Easing the Transition from Curative to Palliative Care

From the patient's perspective, there should be a sense of continuity in care, with a minimum of changes in health care providers. The transition from acute curative care to palliative care should never be an abrupt, traumatic experience. Ideally, patients would be informed of potential outcomes of treatments from the beginning (i.e., whether the treatment is intended for cure or palliation) and the parameters for determining benefits and burdens. The *Oxford Textbook of Palliative Medicine* (Doyle, Hanks, & MacDonald, 1998) offers some helpful guidelines for consideration of disease-modifying therapy. In addition, good symptom management, psychosocial support, and patient autonomy should be a part of care prior to hospice.

Several models have been suggested for cooperative interaction of acute and palliative care. One model identifies four phases of treatment instead of just two (curative and palliative). These four phases are (a) curative, (b) active palliation to prolong life, (c) passive palliation to improve quality of life, and (d) support and comfort care in late-stage disease.

In 1990, the World Health Organization proposed a model in which pain relief and palliative care are part of care from the time of a cancer diagnosis. With the progression of disease, cancer-fighting treatments would gradually decrease as palliative measures increase. Although there are a variety of efforts in this direction in the United States, we are a long way from this ideal.

Clinicians with hospice experience and expertise can help reduce the trauma of transition in several ways:

- Public education to make hospice a familiar concept

- Professional education to help physicians, social workers, nurses, and other professionals in nonhospice settings understand hospice and to suggest how hospice can be presented in a positive way to patients

- Professional education to share palliative care concepts with colleagues in nonhospice settings so these concepts can be integrated earlier in the plan of care

All possible measures should be taken to ensure that patients are involved in decision making to the extent that they wish to be. They need to know it is OK to ask questions and may need encouragement to write down questions of importance to them. They need to know they have the right to be fully informed of their condition and the potential outcomes of treatment options. Clinicians are ethically bound to inform patients of their right to accept or refuse any treatment and to document what their wishes would be when they are unable to speak for themselves. (For further discussion of legal and ethical issues, see chapter 11.)

## Application of Palliative or "Comfort" Care

### Enduring Expert Care

Discontinuing active curative treatment is not synonymous with saying, "There is nothing more to be done." There is always something that can be done for the patient. Palliative care means excellent symptom control by a skilled health care team. Providing enduring expert physical care takes all the resources, science, and knowledge required in acute care but frequently is applied with more intensity and perseverance, and certainly with a different goal in mind: comfort, not cure or correction of abnormal lab values.

The change from cure orientation to comfort orientation automatically implies expertise in relieving distressing symptoms. Because at this point in the patient's history relief of symptoms is a higher priority than the cause of those symptoms, there is less reason for diagnostic studies and traditional interventions, which may cause more distress without any ultimate benefit. This new focus puts us in a different problem-solving paradigm, with different objectives. Rather than measuring the effects of a particular test, medication, or treatment on the disease process, we must measure the benefits and burdens relative to the patient's distress in dying.

### Symptom Management

Every team member, but especially the nurse, must be alert to each new symptom as it appears and adjust care to address it. Keen observation must be made of patient conditions requiring the attention of the physician. It is important to identify when the patient/family is responding appropriately and when it is time to call in some other member of the interdisciplinary team to offer assistance.

The most urgent of distressing symptoms is pain. Unrelieved pain is still a tremendous problem in our health care system, frequently aggravated by ill-reasoned fears of addiction. When a patient is experiencing pain, there is no possibility of working on plans for other physical or psychosocial distresses: The patient is incapable of dealing with anything else when the pain is unrelieved. Hospice, however, has studied and synthesized information to develop effective protocols for pain control with minimal side effects.

The assessment should include not only distressing symptoms that are observed but also any the patient reports as bothersome. Hospice protocols address the amelioration of symptoms, plan for prevention of anticipated symptoms, and anticipate the need for medication for potential "breakthrough" symptoms. Caregivers must pay close attention to body cleanliness, eradication of offensive odors, and any other physical care interventions that will optimize the patient's comfort, function, and self-esteem.

## Spiritual Care

Regardless of the degree or nature of their religious beliefs, most human beings facing death have some basic spiritual distress. This may be as simple as wanting to know that their lives have mattered. The more frequent distresses reported by dying patients are unresolved issues of forgiveness (forgiving or being forgiven), love (to express love or know one is loved), and belonging (need for relationships). At the end of life many people will find themselves returning to an earlier faith or intensely searching for answers about the meaning of life, suffering, and death. These topics will be covered in chapter 7.

Emotional and spiritual pains actually may be greater than patients' physical pains or, at least, may magnify their physical pains. When patients recognize that death is inevitable, spiritual, social, economic, and psychological distresses come sharply into focus, frequently compounding the challenge of effectively managing physical distresses. To obtain comprehensive assessments and effective plans of care, the early pioneers of hospice recognized the absolute necessity for an interdisciplinary team.

## Bereavement

Expert care also includes understanding and accepting the behavior of the grieving patient and the family, no matter how they look, talk, or behave at any given moment. Much overt behavior may be the acting out of frustrations about the loss of control. Interventions must include efforts at restoring a sense of control (e.g., encouraging participation in family plans and decisions, allowing the patient to dispense and administer his or her own medications, establish a plan for treatments or meals, or write a will, if appropriate).

## Availability

An essential part of supportive care of the terminally ill is availability of team members. The patient with unrelieved pain should not have to wait for long periods of time for new orders. If the patient is bleeding, panicked family members need immediate advice about what to do. They need to know they can reach someone, any time of day or night, who can tell them whether or not the symptom is an expected complication and what actions to take. They need to know if a condition is an emergency that can be remedied by professional interventions. Much of the crisis element can be eliminated with on-call nurses, medication orders for anticipated symptoms, and preparation of family members for potential problems. Having the knowledge that someone is available at all times helps the patient and family cope with the situation, provides comfort, and allows the patient to remain at home.

## Continuity

The challenge of providing enduring expert care means that not only will care be comprehensive but that the same plan of care and the same quality of care will continue across settings. This will require interaction among all team members and other agencies, will necessitate the involvement of family and significant others, and will be accompanied by good documentation.

## Medical Expertise

Every hospice names a physician as medical director, who has the responsibility of reviewing all policies and ascertaining an appropriate plan of care for each patient. The medical director also reviews appropriateness of medical eligibility for hospice services and is available to provide primary care to the patient if the patient's attending physician is unable to do so.

## Patient Nonabandonment

Patients often fear being left alone to die. Not only is death one of our greatest fears, it has been made more difficult to confront because of the gradual expulsion of death from common experience in our society. Because of medical advances, children and young adults have decreasing exposure to death and dying. Assuring patients that they and their families will not be abandoned during this unfamiliar and frightening experience can reduce the stress level and aid the adaptive process.

Patients also fear that when they refuse further curative therapies, their physicians will cease to care for them. Unfortunately, studies indicate that the hopelessly ill do receive less attention in the acute hospital setting. Since health care workers at all levels have been indoctrinated with a "cure" orientation and are given little to no preparation to deal with the dying, most do indeed feel very uncomfortable in the presence of such patients. As a result there is a high level of avoidance. Patients are physically isolated by the absence of other people, emotionally isolated when people cannot be open with them, and demoralized when their basic comfort needs are not met. These are all forms of abandonment.

Patients are easily reassured when they are told that someone will be there for them when they have the need. Care providers should strive toward a special sense of "presence" when making a visit. This means going beyond the treatment (e.g., the bath or procedure) to ascertain patients' concerns and to address those concerns. Patients and families will know when caregivers are comfortable just being present with them and walking with them on their difficult journey.

Another way of reassuring and demonstrating your concern as a caregiver for patients and families is thinking ahead with them. For example, this might include calling the next day to see how a new medication is working instead of waiting for someone to call you, initiating anticipatory grief work, preparing the patient and family for possible future events, or observing the progression of ongoing symptoms.

Sometimes it is not just health care workers who are guilty of abandonment; sometimes family members unconsciously do this. Because of the patient's declining energy, performance status, or body image, even those who care will tend to leave the patient out of social events, decisions, or even self-care without realizing they are abandoning or giving up on the person. The hospice team can make a difference by suggesting ways the patient can be included in various family activities and maintain an active part in family life.

## Psychosocial Comfort

Few, if any, of our patients will use terms like *closure, peace of mind,* or *finishing business.* Yet almost every patient will have some emotional, social, or spiritual distress that burns at their inner being and usually expresses itself in anger, frustration, depression, or physical pain.

The emotional or psychological distress observed in patients who are terminally ill is almost always a result of their conscious and subconscious fears, or of their feelings of uselessness and hopelessness. The symptoms exhibited may be anxiety, anger, insomnia, depression, irritability, or physical complaints. The biggest fear in all of us is of death itself, or at least, fear of not knowing what it will feel like, how it will happen, and what to expect next. There are fears of the disease process, how much pain one might have, whether one will be rational, even fears of judgment or punishment in the afterlife. We will probably not remove these fears, but much can be done to improve patients' ability to cope.

The social distresses expressed by dying patients usually involve very basic, practical matters. A husband may be worried about how his wife will manage without him if she has never learned to drive or to write a check. A father may be highly distressed if the potential exists for his family to lose their home without his income. Financial concerns are frequently a major problem, followed closely by legal matters such as wills, ownership, agreements, funeral arrangements, and the like. Loss of job, position, and control are devastating. On a personal level, there is great distress over not being able to function as a father or mother, husband or wife, or community member.

Hospice team members must never expect that they can solve all the problems of dying patients and their families, nor that everyone will die in perfect peace, having made everything right. However, we are responsible for being aware that, for many, this is a final chance for healing, and we must be willing to walk with them on the path they choose.

## Hospice Appropriateness

Hospice is not for everyone. Some patients who are terminally ill will choose to continue aggressive and/or experimental treatments, or ultimately will not wish to talk about their poor prognosis or impending death with anyone. That is their choice. However, as care-givers we have a responsibility to be sure that patients who are referred to us are appropriate candidates for hospice care. When hospice began, only terminal cancer patients were referred for care. Later, hospice began to include people with other diagnoses. This action was appropriate, but it increased the problem of arriving at a prognosis. To help with the problem of prognosis, the National Hospice Organization (1996) has produced a useful monograph entitled *Medical Guidelines for Determining Prognosis in Selected Non-Cancer Diseases*. A physician task force summarized the literature to give us general guidelines for determining limited prognosis (6 months), as well as prognoses for heart disease, pulmonary disease, dementia, HIV disease, liver disease, renal disease, stroke, and amyotrophic lateral sclerosis. The nature of these diseases will be discussed more extensively in chapter 4.

### REFERENCES AND SELECTED READINGS

Bentivegna, J. F. (1992). *When to refuse treatment*. Rocky Hill, CT: Michelle Publishing.

Byock, I. R. (1997). *Dying well: The prospect for growth at the end of life*. New York: Riverhead Books.

Doyle D., Hanks, G. W. C., & MacDonald, N. (Eds.). (1998). *Oxford textbook of palliative medicine* (2nd ed.). New York: Oxford University Press.

Feifel, H. (1977). *New meanings of death.* New York: McGraw-Hill.

Kastenbaum, R., & Aisenberg, R. (1972). *The psychology of death.* New York: Springer.

Kilburn, L. H. (1988). *Hospice operations manual.* South Deerfield, MA: National Hospice Organization.

Kübler-Ross, E. (1969). *On death and dying: What the dying have to teach doctors, nurses, clergy, and their own families.* New York: Macmillan.

Kübler-Ross, E. (1975). *Death: The final stage of growth.* Englewood Cliffs, NJ: Prentice Hall.

Last Acts Task Force on Palliative Care. (1997). *Precepts of palliative care.* Princeton, NJ: Robert Wood Johnson Foundation.

National Hospice Organization. (1993). *Standards of a hospice program of care.* South Deerfield, MA: Author.

National Hospice Organization. (1996). *Medical guidelines for determining prognosis in selected non-cancer diseases* (2nd ed.). South Deerfield, MA: Author.

National Hospice Organization. (1998). *Hospice care: A physician's guide.* South Deerfield, MA: Author.

National Hospice Organization. (1999). *Guide to the nation's hospices, 1998/99.* South Deerfield, MA: Author.

Parkes, C. M. (1996). *Bereavement: Studies of grief in adult life* (3rd ed.). London: Routledge.

Quint, J. C. (1967). *The nurse and the dying patient.* New York: Macmillan.

Saunders, C., Baines, M., & Dunlop, R. (1995). *Living with dying: A guide to palliative care* (3rd ed.). London: Oxford University Press.

Shneidman, E. (1976). *Death: Current perspectives.* Palo Alto, CA: Mayfield.

Stoddard, S. (1992). *The hospice movement: A better way of caring for the dying* (rev. ed.). New York: Vintage Books.

Weisman, A. D. (1972). *On dying and denying: A psychiatric study of terminality.* New York: Behavioral Publications.

World Health Organization. (1990). *Cancer pain relief and palliative care* (Technical Report Series 804). Geneva, Switzerland: Author.

# CHAPTER 2

# The Interdisciplinary Team

**PURPOSE**

The purpose of this chapter is to describe the structure and functions of an interdisciplinary hospice team in the delivery of palliative care to hospice patients.

**OBJECTIVES**

Upon completion of this chapter, the learner will be able to:

1. Identify the major difference between multidisciplinary and interdisciplinary teams

2. Describe the roles and responsibilities of team members

3. Describe regularly scheduled team care-plan meetings and the value of total team involvement

**CONTENT OUTLINE**

   I. Value of the Interdisciplinary Team

  II. Team Roles

     A. Physicians

     B. Nurses

     C. Social workers

     D. Clergy

     E. Therapists

     F. Other consultative disciplines

     G. Volunteers

## VALUE OF THE INTERDISCIPLINARY TEAM

The interdisciplinary team (IDT) is fundamental to comprehensive hospice care. *Interdisciplinary,* as opposed to *multidisciplinary,* implies that team members do not work in isolation but participate in an ongoing team process of assessing and planning. Throughout the process, the approach to medical, nursing, psychosocial, or spiritual problems is enriched by input from all the disciplines represented on the team. The hospice professional works in consort with other team members, reflecting a unified team approach, developed at regularly scheduled meetings. For many hospices, meetings are scheduled on a weekly basis. The hospice team manifests a mutual respect for the value and unique expertise of each discipline yet accepts the need for flexibility and overlap of roles. For example, a patient who is afraid or worried about finances may exhibit anger about meals or translate the distress to physical pain. The doctor, nurse, social worker, volunteer, or any other team member may detect this transference and raise it as a treatment issue.

The successful functioning of the hospice IDT can be maximized when there is a clear philosophy pertaining to palliative care and ethical issues, open intrateam and team/family communications, flexible leadership, and willingness to deal with differences. Staff expertise in systems management and in psychosocial/spiritual issues will be enhanced through the provision of, or access to, inservice educational programs for the team as a whole, as well as for members of specific disciplines.

## TEAM ROLES

Following is a brief outline of the key disciplines often found on a hospice IDT. Each program will need to determine its own specific needs in terms of team membership. Regardless of team composition, each team member must understand and appreciate the philosophy and objectives of the hospice program and respect and utilize the strengths and skills of other team members.

## Physicians

The hospice physician orchestrates the treatments and gives the medical orders that will most effectively ameliorate distressing symptoms. This challenging role applies all the knowledge gained in acute medicine to palliative care goals. The hospice physician contributes much strength and support to the team effort with knowledge of disease processes and trajectories, appropriate interventions, and confirmation of team plans. The hospice physician will interact with other team members, the patient, the patient's family, and the patient's attending physician to coordinate the most effective plan of care.

## Nurses

Nurses play a major role in hospice care because they are the team members who spend the most time with patients and who are responsible for ongoing assessment and planning for immediate care needs. Nurses must be astute at assessing patients' verbal and nonverbal messages related to every aspect of physical and emotional comfort. They must be mindful of preventive actions (e.g., preventing decubiti or constipation), and they must remember to include the family in assessment, teaching, and support.

## Social Workers

The psychosocial problems that emerge with a life-threatening illness can be immense. The social worker assesses and plans interventions for financial concerns, family matters, grief, and environmental problems. The social worker is involved with therapeutic counseling, identifying community resources, and assisting the team in understanding the patient's and family's psychosocial problems and coping patterns.

## Clergy

The spiritual professional plays a primary role in addressing and coordinating the spiritual and religious needs of the patient and family. The hospice chaplain may be the sole spiritual caregiver or may assist in arranging for involvement of family clergy. The chaplain must be open to a wide variety of values and beliefs but recognize that almost everyone has inner thoughts that can result in distress of the spirit. The chaplain may also be active in staff support and/or the bereavement program.

## Therapists

Physical therapists, occupational therapists, music therapists, and so on contribute a great deal to the comfort and quality of life of the dying patient. They may hold the key to increased mobility and independence, which can be of utmost importance to the patient and the family. They are also skilled at interventions for pain problems and poor mental outlook.

### Other Consultative Disciplines

Patients with end-stage disease often have multisystem failure and are on a large number of medications. *Pharmacists* can suggest effective drug regimens with reduced risk of adverse interactions or excretion problems. They can contribute to knowledge of analgesics and proper dosing. Since eating problems occur with great frequency in terminally ill patients, input from *dietitians* can be very helpful. Like all team members, dietitians must view the patient from the palliative care perspective and suggest ways in which nutrition can be comforting, as opposed to optimizing nutritional status. They can suggest interventions that are individualized to the patient's food preferences, swallowing capacity, and metabolic/mechanical gastrointestinal discomforts. Mental health practitioners such as *psychiatrists* and *psychologists* can play a valuable role in both direct patient care and staff support. In addition to offering treatment for patient symptoms, they may strengthen the staff by bolstering their coping skills when necessary and by providing advice on handling difficult patient/family dilemmas.

### Volunteers

Volunteers are an essential component of hospice care. Not only are they a valuable part of the team, they are required under Medicare. Like other team members, volunteers must be carefully selected and trained for hospice. In particular, volunteers should not be on the team to work out their own feelings of grief or guilt. Volunteers will have a variety of talents: Some may perform tasks in the patient's home, whereas others may want to do errands or office work. The tasks will vary, but all will be valuable contributions to the overall success of the program. Some possible volunteer assignments are listed in Table 2.1. Volunteer orientation should include an overview of the hospice program and its philosophy, some basic communication skills (e.g., active listening and nonjudgmental attitude), confidentiality requirements, and safety and emergency issues.

## SELECTION AND TRAINING OF HOSPICE STAFF

Dr. Jack Zimmerman of Church Hospital Hospice in Baltimore, Maryland, suggests that a hospice program is only as good as its individual staff members (Zimmerman & Roche, 1986). The important qualities to look for are competence, sensitivity, flexibility, maturity,

## Table 2.1   Ideas for Volunteer Assignments

PHYSICAL CARE

> Assisting with meals or snacks
>
> Patient care, bath, bed
>
> Observation, safety

PSYCHOSOCIAL CARE

> Active listening, companionship
>
> Reading, writing, escort activities
>
> Diversions, hobbies, crafts, music
>
> Life celebrations, holiday activities, parties

AESTHETICS

> Housekeeping, hospitality
>
> Flowers, home atmosphere, hairdressing, shaving

STAFF SUPPORT

> Phone, messages, clerical
>
> Errands, projects

BEREAVEMENT

> Addressing sympathy cards
>
> Wakes, funerals, family calls

and spirituality. He broadly defines *spirituality* as inner strength and openness to finding meaning in life. Hospice teacher, author, and researcher Dr. Madalon Amenta (1984) studied the traits of hospice nurses and identified them to be significantly more assertive, imaginative, forthright, freethinking, and independent than their colleagues in other practice settings. The experience of most hospice programs suggests that these two lists of qualities can be combined as shown in Table 2.2. Background, experience, and age are not as important as a positive, flexible, and responsible outlook. It is unnecessary for team members to be completely resolved about death, especially their own; rather, they should be able to be honest about what they feel and open to other people's values and fears.

The training of new staff members varies according to their previous experience and disciplines, but it should include an overview that will sensitize all disciplines to the roles of other team members and to the overall goals and challenges of participating on a team caring for dying patients.

---

## Table 2.2    Desirable Traits for Hospice Staff

*Flexibility* in handling complex situations with patients, families, and staff who may frequently be under a great deal of stress from grief and upheaval

*Autonomy* to make independent decisions with competence and confidence, and to assume responsibility for actions taken

*Sensitivity* to the values and belief systems of a wide variety of peoples and cultures, and in acquiring good judgment in responses

*Openness* to new ideas, new information, new approaches (i.e., involvement of family and team), and to differing opinions

*Spirituality,* which results in a respect for self and others, and recognition of the value of belief systems and meaning

---

# INTERDISCIPLINARY CARE PLANNING

## Collaboration

Collaboration implies the sharing of information and ideas for a common goal. In hospice care, it means sharing information and opinions among other disciplines, as well as from volunteers, patients, and family members. Hospice is an approach that is truly holistic, with input from a variety of disciplines, and truly individualized for each patient, by virtue of its openness to patient/family values.

Collaboration not only serves the patient's best interests, it also strengthens individual team members. This occurs through mutual sharing of knowledge as well as interaction about group process and organization. The collaborative group setting provides caregivers an opportunity to process feelings of loss and to receive support on an ongoing basis.

## Plan of Care

Planning begins on the patient's admission visit and is developed by the team into a comprehensive plan of care within 48 hours. At regularly scheduled meetings, care plans are evaluated for effectiveness. This review includes consideration of symptom protocols in use, as well as psychosocial and spiritual interventions. It is important also to evaluate the disease trajectory (the rapidity and complexity of the disease course) on a regular basis because the focus of care often changes as the patient draws closer to death. New problems or situations requiring intervention usually become apparent as patient and family share more intimate concerns after developing a trusting relationship with team members. A checklist for the care plan review would include the following items:

+ Effectiveness of symptom management

+ Disease trajectory

+ Patient/family psychosocial needs

+ Spiritual needs

## STAFF SUPPORT AND TEAM BUILDING

### Staff Support

Hospice caregivers are at high risk for physical and emotional symptoms of stress due to daily reminders of death, numerous other losses, and perhaps an accompanying sense of failure or helplessness. Regularly, caregivers are forced to face their own mortality, and they may not be comfortable with that knowledge. Health care workers are generally attuned to making people better and seeing "happy endings." Even when team members accept the inevitability of death, they still may berate themselves when patients die without having resolved personal or interpersonal conflicts.

The IDT plays a vital role in preventing burnout among its members. The team must practice openness to individual opinion, sensitivity to personal feelings, and balance between seriousness and humor. Table 2.3 presents some ideas for preventing staff burnout.

### Team Building

It is inevitable that a group of people who work closely together will have differing viewpoints that can ultimately result in conflicts. Recognizing this, and planning to deal with conflicts within the team, results in increased productivity and effectiveness. Refusal to deal with team conflicts, or the inability to resolve them, leads to increased interpersonal problems and diminished team effectiveness.

Dr. Dale Larson, noted clinical psychologist and consultant, has presented some useful and practical guidelines for an effective caregiving team and, specifically, for conflict resolution (Larson, 1993). He stresses that honest and open communication can prevent the development of serious problems, simply through the processes of clarifying and sharing. He also stresses the importance of conflict resolution without personalizing problems or undermining other team members' self-esteem. The productive and effective team plans measures proactively; it does not wait for a crisis and then react.

## Table 2.3  Ideas for Preventing Burnout

*Ongoing education,* so staff feel confident and validated in their jobs

*Openness,* so conflicts and disagreements are dealt with, not ignored

*Sensitivity* to recognize when someone is having a bad day and needs space or emotional support

*Staff support meetings or retreats* to permit sharing, affirming one another, and addressing special issues of concern

*Encouragement* of professional growth toward being a "facilitator" rather than a "solver" of all problems

*Planned humor breaks,* undertaking (in a sensitive way) specific projects or activities to recognize the humorous and amusing side of life

*Mechanisms for positive feedback,* so all staff members are aware of appreciation

*Acknowledgment of grief* as a legitimate response in a team member, particularly if there was a special bonding to a particular patient or family

In his book *Overextended and Undernourished,* Dennis Portnoy (1996) emphasizes how important it is for individuals in helping roles to take responsibility for their own self-care. He warns of self-imposed stresses, such as exaggerating one's own responsibility, absorbing other people's feelings and problems, and maintaining a "peace at any price" attitude. He suggests routine evaluation of self-care and a plan of action for personal nurturing to maintain healthy mental and physical functioning.

In summary, to achieve the goal of optimal physical, spiritual, and psychosocial comfort for the patient/family, the team must work at strengthening the group process. Team building does not just happen. It requires a concentrated effort to learn effective means of conflict resolution, to establish mechanisms for feedback, to practice open communication, and to recognize the need for educational or support meetings.

### REFERENCES AND SUGGESTED READINGS

Adams, J. P., Hershatter, M. J., & Moritz, D. A. (1991). Accumulated loss phenomenon among hospice caregivers. *American Journal of Hospice and Palliative Care,* 8(3), 29–37.

Amenta, M. O. (1984). Traits of hospice nurses compared with those who work in traditional settings. *Journal of Clinical Psychology, 40*(2), 414–420.

Foster, Z., & Davidson, K. W. (1995). Satisfactions and stresses for the social worker. In I. B. Corless, B. G. Germino, & M. A. Pittman (Eds.), *A challenge for living.* Boston: Jones and Bartlett.

Hull, M. M. (1991). Hospice nurses: Caring support for caregiving families. *Cancer Nursing, 14*(2), 63–70.

Larson D. G. (1993). *The helper's journey: Working with people facing grief, loss, and life-threatening illness.* Champaign, IL: Research Press.

Lentz, R. J., & Ramsey, L. F. (1988). The psychologist consultant on the hospice team: One example of the model. *The Hospice Journal, 4*(2), 55–66.

Meade, V. (1991). A pharmacist helps dying patients. *American Pharmacy, NS31*(10), 49–52.

Parry, J. K. (1989). *Social work theory and practice with the terminally ill.* Binghamton, NY: Haworth.

Portnoy, D. (1996). *Overextended and undernourished.* Minneapolis: Johnson Institute.

Vachon, M. L. S. (1987). *Occupational stress in the care of the critically ill, the dying and the bereaved.* Washington, DC: Hemisphere.

Vachon, M. L. S. (1989). Team stress in palliative/hospice care. *The Hospice Journal, 3*(2/3), 75–103.

Zimmerman, J. M., & Roche, K. A. (1986). The hospice care team. In J. M. Zimmerman & K. A. Roche (Eds.), *Hospice: Complete care of the terminally ill.* Baltimore: Urban and Schwarzenberg.

# CHAPTER 3

# Family Dynamics and Therapeutic Communication

**PURPOSE**

The purpose of this chapter is to explore the elements of family assessment and to heighten awareness of therapeutic versus nontherapeutic communication.

**OBJECTIVES**

After completing this chapter, the learner will be able to:

1. List four elements of family assessment

2. Identify at least three procedures of care frequently taught to the caregiver

3. Discuss some of the major differences between therapeutic and nontherapeutic communication

**CONTENT OUTLINE**

I. Assessing the Family Unit

   A. Relationships and roles

   B. Coping patterns

   C. Specific resource information and educational deficits

   D. Cultural and ethnic implications

II. Principles of Therapeutic Communication

   A. Techniques of interacting

   B. Active listening

C.  Facilitator role

D.  Therapeutic versus nontherapeutic responses

# ASSESSING THE FAMILY UNIT

## Relationships and Roles

The reason we assess the patient and family as a unit is that every family group has developed its own unique patterns of interacting and reacting. The intricacies of the operating dynamics of the family system impact how family members cope and develop, either as individuals or collectively. Therefore, to be an effective facilitator it is necessary to evaluate what those dynamics are. Whereas individual family members may have different points of view as adults, they all share common history, losses, and family stories.

Assessing the family system cannot be done in one visit. By observing and interacting over time, it usually becomes apparent who plays what roles: a caring role, a dominant role, a detached role, and so forth. A genogram can be helpful in expediting the evaluation process. A genogram is like a family tree but also shows relationships and elicits coping responses. (For a sample genogram, see Kaye, 1990).

Some common terms used in describing family systems are as follows:

+ *Open family system:* One in which there are open communications, predictability, interdependence, and interactions with entities outside the family. The opposite would be the *closed family system,* in which the family interacts primarily among its own members. Families go back and forth between closed and open, but staying closed is an unhealthy coping mechanism.

+ *Enmeshed family system:* This system exhibits power struggles and attempts to control its members and is characterized by loss of personal autonomy for individuals. The opposite would be the *disengaged family system,* in which family members are usually distant, have infrequent contacts, have rigid boundaries, and are emotionally disconnected.

+ *Differentiated family system:* This family system exhibits healthy separateness and independence.

Personality traits also have a bearing on family interactions and outcomes. For example, an introverted patient may depend on an extroverted family member to be the liaison between the home and outside professionals and agencies. This can present problems if the spokesperson is insensitive to or in disagreement with the patient's values and priorities. Team members may not be able to change who the spokesperson is, but awareness of such difficulties may help in planning ways to expedite the patient's wishes.

It is important to be aware of the stress levels of various family members. During the stress of a patient's terminal diagnosis and diminished functioning, the family unit is likely to experience upheaval and a redistribution of roles. Someone else in the family might now have to take on the role of wage earner, homemaker, and so on. These changes often result in an increased stress level for everyone.

## Coping Patterns

People seldom use only one coping strategy, and it is unlikely that they will always cope in exactly the same way in different situations. Although general patterns of coping can be recognized, expect to see variations depending on concurrent stressors, history of previous losses, and individual experiences of understanding and enlightenment. The key to being therapeutic with different families is to facilitate their own self-assessment and problem solving. *There is no one correct way to cope!*

Table 3.1 outlines some common coping strategies. Some are effective and some are ineffective in achieving desired outcomes, depending on the severity of the problem. In general, people look for the least demanding solution (a "quick fix"), rather than use strategies that may be more painful but that render better long-term results. Therapeutic approaches to identify coping patterns and to facilitate problem solving include the following:

- Suggest that the problems be clearly defined and prioritized.

- Ascertain if information is available to define the problem accurately.

- Encourage open discussion of potential solutions or outcomes; this may help in setting goals.

- Lead or facilitate a patient/family meeting, but remember, ways of coping must come from family members, either collectively or individually.

## Specific Resource Information and Educational Deficits

If hospice team members try to perform all necessary physical care and take care of all social issues, the patient and family can become increasingly dependent and less able to cope with any new developments. A more therapeutic and helpful approach is to provide neces-

## Table 3.1   Common Coping Strategies

1. Confront the problem and take appropriate actions.
2. Deny as much as possible.
3. Conform and comply with what is expected or advised.
4. Seek out information and direction.
5. Resign yourself to what cannot be changed.
6. Forget about it and think of other things.
7. Keep busy with interests or new pursuits unrelated to the problem.
8. Share concerns with interested or experienced persons.
9. Do something, anything; even if futile, it shows effort.
10. Redefine the problem and look for realistic possibilities.
11. Release emotional tension by venting your feelings.
12. Retreat from the problem or postpone dealing with it.
13. Review alternatives, rationally reflecting on the consequences.
14. Laugh it off and change the subject.
15. Blame or shame someone or something; that places responsibility outside yourself.

sary information and encouragement to facilitate patient and family independence and coping. Some common areas requiring this therapeutic approach are summarized in Table 3.2.

### Social Concerns

Families who have experienced major or long-term medical care may be financially depleted. If, in addition, the patient was the person whose job provided the majority of the income, the family may find themselves in very difficult financial straits. Issues of wills, insurance, or other legal matters may require the help of legal advisors. Team members, volunteers, or members of the family network all may be resources for such things as helping a patient's spouse learn how to drive, how to balance a checkbook, or how to seek out a job or job training. However, when professional and specialized services are indicated, the hospice team should be aware of available community programs, including mental health and social service agencies, transportation services, legal assistance, and so forth.

### Safety Issues

Preventing falls or injuries to weakened or confused patients should include plans for walkers, wheelchairs, bathroom aids, hospital beds,

## Table 3.2   Areas Requiring Information and Education

*Social concerns:* Financial problems, personal/legal documents, new skills, transportation

*Safety issues:* Ambulation, driving, self-dosing, lifting, transferring

*Caregiver skills:* Recognizing disease processes and potential complications, understanding proper use and side effects of medications, learning and practicing specific procedures (ostomy, tracheotomy, wounds, etc.)

*Crisis events:* Hemorrhage, severe dyspnea, mental status changes, death

*Emotional and spiritual care:* Value of expression, recognizing and managing stress, setting realistic goals, identifying supports

side rails, and the like. For the caregiver and the patient, instructions on proper use of equipment, lifting and transfer techniques, and specific safety issues are essential. Some particular safety issues relate to smoking around oxygen tanks or placement of furniture in the home. The team may need to get involved if the patient continues to drive although he or she becomes physically or mentally impaired to the point of being unsafe behind the wheel.

### Caregiver Skills

Though some family caregivers may never be able to manage specific procedures such as bathing, tube feeding, open wound care, or suctioning a tracheotomy, with some instruction, practice, reinforcement, and support most will find that they can do more than they thought possible. Their understanding of the disease process and potential complications will enhance their abilities. This information may not need to be provided in great detail, but it should be enough for them to understand what distress the disease is causing the patient and what can be done to relieve that distress. In particular, they need instruction in the proper administration of medication, as well as about potential side effects and interactions.

### Crisis Events

*Crisis* means different things to different people. The more the patient and family caregivers are informed about a condition, its symptoms and management, and available resources, the less likely they will be to make panic calls. Family caregivers need to know they can call someone in the hospice program at any time to seek reassurance that they are doing the right thing. This reassurance may prevent escalation to a panic situation or a hospital admission.

The crises that commonly cause panic calls to hospice or emergency-care staff are severe pain, anxiety attack, dyspnea (inability to get sufficient air), hemorrhage, wild behavior, convulsions, and death. For all of these, a discussion and mental rehearsal ahead of time may prevent futile emergency intervention or inappropriate hospital admissions. For example, if a patient has an extensive head and neck cancer encroaching on the carotid arteries, family caregivers should be informed that severe hemorrhage is highly possible, that the situation is not preventable or reversible, and that it can be the cause of death. Most hospices suggest having dark towels or sheets available to compress the area and to minimize the traumatic sight of gross bleeding. Part of caregiver preparation is relaying the value of remaining calm and reassuring to the patient. With dyspnea, caregivers will need training and support to develop needed skills to know the medications, environment, and interactions that are effective as opposed to those that could worsen the condition. Preparing caregivers ahead of time greatly enhances their ability to cope with crisis events.

### Emotional and Spiritual Care

Patients and family caregivers will need education to recognize symptoms of and techniques for managing stress, as well as encouragement to indulge in caring for themselves. This last may mean periods of rest or respite away from the patient for physical and emotional rejuvenation. Caregivers may need guidance in setting realistic goals; often unrealistic goals indicate a need for more accurate information. Identification of available support networks will help family members help themselves. These support networks often are other family members, neighbors, friends, clubs, or church groups. It is important to recognize when emotional or spiritual distresses among the family are beyond the scope of the team and when referrals to mental health professionals or spiritual leaders should be made.

## Cultural and Ethnic Implications

The ethnicity of the patient/family will often bear upon treatment decisions and the therapeutic impact of the plan of care. In fact, knowing the particulars of customs related to food, hygiene, and health care among certain ethnic and religious groups can be essential to establishing a good plan of care. Knowing patient/family perceptions of positive or negative caring behaviors likewise will result in more effective interactions. Awareness of the rituals and beliefs related to the circumstances before, during, and after the death event will assist the team in comforting the family and in avoiding religious and cultural faux pas.

Death is the final life transition for all human beings, but in each culture, and in each family within a culture, specific practices will hold meaning and be essential to grief resolution. Following is a brief summary of some beliefs in some of the major ethnic groups. These are generalizations, and the responses of particular families or individuals within these groups may vary widely. Variations frequently also occur as groups or individuals become acculturated to the customs of the country to which they have relocated.

### Chinese/Asian

In contrast to Western medicine, which in large part has a scientific or organic view of most diseases, medicine in China and other Asian cultures reflects a more holistic concept. Asian peoples generally view illness as resulting from physical, metaphysical, and supernatural elements. They perceive mind and body as inseparable and illness as a result of imbalance or disharmony within the self, or as the self interacts with the environment. They may be reluctant to agree to testing, medications, or surgery, preferring their traditional methods of herbs, acupuncture, or other ways of regaining the balance of the life forces.

Asian peoples are remarkably tenacious, and most have a stoic reaction to pain. They value equanimity and will withdraw rather than complain. Personal feelings, decisions, and interactions are generally kept within the family, with males having the dominant role. These patients would be unlikely to discuss the details of an illness or their reactions to it.

Although there is a wide range in religions and beliefs, many Asian people are strongly guided by the "spirit world," worshipping ancestors or believing in reincarnation. Pleasing the spirits is important because that may influence one's experience in the next life. For this reason, it is helpful to ascertain the religious and funeral rituals important to the family and find ways to assist them in carrying these out.

### Jewish

The Jewish faith views death as inevitable but highly honors life and the sacredness of the body (a divine gift). Jewish people would be unlikely to perform any action that might shorten human life, including discussion of imminent death or crying in the patient's presence if they thought doing so would diminish hope and therefore hasten death. For the dying person, it is a time for confessions and blessings. For the friends and family, it is a time for honoring the dying person, attending to the patient's comfort, showing respect, and offering the support of their presence. The patient is never left alone; it is important that someone be present when the soul separates from the body.

Ritual washing and continual watch honor the body of the dead. A plain casket is used, there is no cremation, and autopsy is opposed. The body is buried within 24 hours without the usual embalming and cosmetics common to the funeral practices of many other groups in the United States.

Judaism has prescribed laws that acknowledge normal grief reaction and involve the community in comforting mourners. The designated grief periods are Shiva, 30 days of readjustment, and 11 months of remembrance. Shiva is a 7-day period of withdrawing from usual activities to allow for grieving. During this time, family and friends visit to remember the deceased. The remainder of the first 30 days is still a period of adjustment, but normal activities are resumed. On the 1-year anniversary, a special memorial service, Yahrzeit, is held.

## Native American

Similar to Asian peoples, Native Americans believe that the body, mind, and spirit are integrally linked. They also believe that the spirits of the dead influence the living and that the spirit of someone deceased will reside where the person died. Except for the Navajo, most nations believe in an afterlife. They see birth and death as sacred events and the lifetime in between as an opportunity to live well and show kindness, both to others and to the environment. The body is respected, and cremation is not usually performed.

Because this group generally accepts death as a natural and expected event, denial, anger, and expressions of grief usually are minimal. A death is considered a family event. There will be extensive family and community gathering to honor the dead and support the mourners. A remembrance is kept, such as a lock of hair (or in modern times, a picture) to remind loved ones during the year of mourning to strive for virtuous behavior.

## Spanish-Speaking

As is the case for the other groups discussed, Spanish-speaking people are not a monolithic group; rather, they represent a wide range of cultures: Spanish, Latin American, Mexican, Puerto Rican, and others. However, they are very often of the Catholic faith and view death as a natural part of life. It is important for dying persons to receive last rites or prayers from priests. There are usually large family gatherings, and mourners are often highly emotional in the face of pain, sorrow, or grief. Mourners are comforted by prayers, the lighting of candles, and the open expression of their grief.

# PRINCIPLES OF THERAPEUTIC COMMUNICATION

## Techniques of Interacting

*Therapeutic communication* refers to human interactions in which feelings, values, and information are exchanged toward a beneficial effect. In our interactions with terminally ill patients and the significant people in their lives, this therapeutic effect happens when we successfully identify and facilitate optimal strategies without interjecting personal opinion or judgment. Following are some of the basic principles of therapeutic interaction.

### Get beyond physical distress

Picking up and following through on cues from the patient/family are the most effective ways to ascertain inner fears, emotional distress, and other problems. Usually, the patient or family give cues that they are ready and want to obtain information or share their feelings. If such cues are not forthcoming, it may be therapeutic to encourage open expression. If there is adequate time, it is best to build the bridge of a trusting relationship first. If time seems short, the following phrases may be helpful in encouraging expressions of inner distress:

- "How are your spirits today?"

- "How do you feel within yourself?"

- "What concerns you most right now?"

- "You seem to be in deep thought . . ."

### Do not avoid the reality of what is happening

Dr. Elisabeth Kübler-Ross, who wrote volumes on work with dying patients, teaches us that we should not be concerned about the patient's tolerance for "the truth." Rather, our question should be "Which truth?" She says the question should not be "Should we tell?" Instead, the question should be "How do I share this with my patient?" (Kübler-Ross, 1969, p. 28).

Dr. Avery Weisman, another pioneer in understanding the needs of dying patients, states that patients should know enough to make an informed decision (Weisman, 1984). He also believes the issue is not *if* the patient is told, but *how* it is done. He observes that imagined fear of the unknown is often worse than the reality and that knowledge can reduce the fear of the unknown and correct misperceptions.

If you cannot, or think you should not, answer patients' questions about the illness or prognosis, let them know this and offer to help them put their questions in writing for the doctor. It helps the doctor to have questions clearly stated, and it helps the patients or family remember the questions if they are written down. This process also gives other members of the team a better idea of what information patients desire or feel they need.

### Permit denial, but do not support false hopes

It is normal and common for people to use denial as a defense in the early stages after hearing bad news. It usually means they need time to digest the information they have been given, repeated input, and information delivered in small increments. If they opt for denial after this point, they can sometimes deal with reality if it is put in a third-person or "what if" context. If patients choose to remain in denial as their way of coping, their decision should be honored. However, this does not mean that clinicians should concur with unrealistic goals or support false information. Some patients may never be able to admit openly that they are dying or that they know they cannot be cured. Even so, they may proceed to take care of necessary business, indicating their inner awareness. Many people need guidance to think in terms of realistic, attainable goals, then encouragement to concentrate on those.

### Encourage expression of feelings

We in the helping professions are accustomed to "fixing things," making everything all right. But for terminally ill patients, everything is not all right. It is natural for them to express their feelings, often demonstrated as tears of despair or screams of anger. Being present and letting patients know it is OK to cry or scream is therapeutic. Reactive depression, crying, and anger are normal responses to massive disappointment and actual or anticipated loss.

### Allow the patient to be in control

When the patient is losing control of many things, including life itself, it is important to let him or her control the parameters of terminal care. Asking a patient what he or she wants, however, is inappropriate if the person is not first informed of options and their potential outcomes. Explore issues the patient *can* control, such as physical arrangement of the home environment, what and when to eat, activity schedule, level of pain to be tolerated, and so forth. Allow the patient to take part in meetings that include future planning for survivors. After needed information has been provided, the following may be helpful in eliciting goals from the patient and family:

- ◆ "Tell me your goals so we will know how best to help you." (If the patient responds, "My goal is to get well," you might say, "And if that isn't possible, then what would your goals be?")

◆ "We want you to tell us how we can best help you. What things are important to you?"

### Assess readiness to receive new information

People usually do not hear or incorporate what they are not ready to hear. It is important to consider how receptive a patient is before attempting to teach that person about the disease process—or any other aspect of the dying experience. You may need to bring an issue to the person's attention and suggest some options, then wait for a response.

### Repeat information as necessary

People who are tired, upset, in pain, or in emotional overload frequently do not remember what they have been told. So, whether explaining a new medication or sharing bad news about the illness, plan to repeat information on another visit and/or leave printed material when appropriate.

### Encourage celebration of life

Don't presume that the patient or family members should always be thinking about the disease and approaching death. While these thoughts may never totally go away, the patient and family may need to talk about mundane life events, celebrate holidays, or simply do things that bring them pleasure. Reassure them that this is normal and acceptable.

## Active Listening

*Active listening* may be defined as honest and compassionate interaction that permits the speaker to coordinate thoughts and to express concerns and fears. It means listening for the other person's agenda, not presenting yours. It means demonstrating a receptive and non-judgmental attitude. Following are some suggestions for being a good listener.

### Assume a "listening" position

Sitting down at the patient's level with nothing in your hands gives a totally different impression than standing at the foot of the bed with chart and pen in hand. If your purpose truly is to hear what the other person's concerns are, as opposed to furthering your own agenda, it will be readily apparent. Eye contact lets the other person know you are not avoiding, or feeling uncomfortable with, what is being said. However, be aware that some individuals may be uncomfortable with direct eye contact.

### Do not presume to know a patient's needs

Being open to another person means letting go of your own precon-
ceived ideas. Being open allows another person's definition of a problem and that person's priorities and usual coping behaviors to
emerge. It also means being open to how much "help" a person needs
or wants. Be aware when the message changes, as may be the case
especially during periods of declining physical or emotional status.
Do not be surprised if the individual's most pressing concern has
nothing to do with the illness or impending death.

### Do not be afraid of silence

If you are talking, you are not listening. If you are talking, you are
probably telling the person what to do or what to think. If you are
talking, you are not allowing the patient to ruminate. If you are not
talking but continue to be present, the patient will know you care and
that what he or she is thinking is more important than what you are
thinking. Silence is OK; we are just not used to it.

### Be aware of nonverbal communication

A quizzical expression of doubt, a frown of disagreement, a serene
smile at something that brings pleasure, an angry face and attitude,
and so forth can be deeply communicative. Pointing out obvious feelings, such as "You look happy about that" or "You seem very angry
today," is quite acceptable.

### Be aware of indirect communication

The patient or family may be unable to face a concern as it relates to
them but may describe it in the third person, as the concern of
"someone they know." Let them stay on safe territory and continue in
the third person.

### Allow the other person to lead the conversation

Do not suggest how or what patient and family need to think.
Therapeutic leads or rephrasing, not interpreting or judging, may
facilitate the expression of their thoughts. Some examples follow:

- "I gather that . . ."
- "If I'm hearing you correctly, you think that . . ."
- "In other words . . ."
- "So you feel that . . ."
- "From your experience, you think . . ."
- "You believe . . ."
- "I wonder if you're saying . . ."

## Facilitator Role

In the facilitator role, one seeks to optimize the other person's coping capacity, not to offer solutions. Facilitating is not only the most therapeutic approach, it prevents the burnout seen in health care professionals who think they must come up with a solution to every problem. The effective facilitator will provide needed information, be available, assist in defining and prioritizing problems, set boundaries, and disavow personal guilt.

### Provide needed information

Often the patient or family members will already know the answers to their own questions but simply need guidance in verbalizing them. At other times, it may be obvious that more information is needed to reach an informed decision. Provision of information about the illness may be in order, or printed information about treatments, medications, and the like may be useful. If there are questions the physician must answer, you can assist the patient and family in writing them out. If the information involves the illness or prognosis, the following inquiries might help open the conversation:

- "What has the doctor told you about your illness?"
- "Share with me how your condition was explained to you."
- "What do you think is happening?"

### Be available

Impress on the patient and family that they can talk with any team member about any question or concern. Just knowing someone will be available and responsive can ease anxiety.

Assist in defining and prioritizing problems. As you are listening to the patient or family express concerns and fears, assimilate and organize the information to help them establish a problem list, priorities, and feasible options. The emotion-laden patient and family will benefit from the views of an objective third person who can separate fact from fancy, help them hear their own words, and condense the issues into manageable problems. Effective ways to clarify issues are repeating, paraphrasing, reflecting, and summarizing what has been said. Hearing one's own thoughts reflected often stimulates redefinition or clarification.

### Set boundaries

Consciously become aware of the limitations of both the agency for which you work and yourself as an individual. Be clear about what is possible and what is not. Observe suffering and respond compassionately, but do not assume personal ownership of the problems and do not encourage patient or family dependence upon you. Set boundaries internally to prevent overinvolvement or identification—both can result in poor judgment or burnout. Doing so will also help to prevent working out one's own agenda or unfinished business.

### Disavow guilt

Consciously disavow guilt on behalf of yourself, the patient, and the family members. You are not responsible for the patient's life situation or belief system. Blaming yourself, or someone else, is nonproductive and wastes energy. The effective facilitator recognizes that no individual is responsible for the patient's illness, unsuccessful treatment, or mortal condition. The challenge is to deal with the tangible realities and feasible coping options for each unique patient and family. Not every patient will choose to finish business, permit comfort, or die peacefully; accept this as inevitable, not as a personal failure.

## Therapeutic versus Nontherapeutic Responses

Many people avoid dying patients and those in grief because they feel they do not know what to say. Certain expressions of pain and confusion are quite common, and it is important to respond to these therapeutically. Table 3.3 lists some of these expressions and some possible responses. Remember, however, that it is perfectly acceptable just to be present without offering any advice at all. Do not be afraid to say, "I don't have any answers, but I'm willing to be here for you."

## Table 3.3  Therapeutic versus Nontherapeutic Responses

| PATIENT/FAMILY EXPRESSION OR REACTION | NONTHERAPEUTIC RESPONSES | THERAPEUTIC RESPONSES |
|---|---|---|
| "I think I'm going to die." | "Now, don't talk like that. Everything is going to be OK." | "Do you feel that bad?"<br>"Why are you thinking about that?"<br>"What is your biggest concern about that?"<br>"Is that what you've been told?" |
| "Why is God doing this to me?" | "God is the last one you should be angry with." | "You think God is causing your illness?" (The patient may not want an answer as much as he or she needs to express anger at what cannot be controlled.) |
| Lashing out angrily at family or staff | "You shouldn't be angry."<br>"Why are you being so unreasonable?" | "You seem to be very angry."<br>"What makes you the most angry?" |
| Expressions of hopelessness and helplessness (despair) | "Now, now, let's look at the bright side."<br>"I know exactly how you feel." | "It's normal to have these emotions." (Or discuss some things the patient *can* control.) |
| "What would you do in my situation?" | "What you should do is . . ."<br>"You need to . . ." | "What options do you have?"<br>"How have you coped with similar problems in the past?" |
| Crying | "Don't cry. Things will get better."<br>"Don't cry. You need to be strong right now." | "It's OK to cry."<br>"It's natural for you to feel like crying; let it out." |
| Screaming out | "Now, don't be upset, calm down and think this through rationally." | "It's OK to let your emotions out." |

41

## REFERENCES AND SUGGESTED READINGS

Amadeo, D. M. (1993). Hospice nurses and approaching death. *American Journal of Hospice and Palliative Care, 10(5)*, 10–12.

Byock, I. R. (1997). *Dying well: The prospect for growth at the end of life.* New York: Riverhead Books.

Buckman, R. (1992). *How to break bad news: A guide for health care professionals.* Baltimore: Johns Hopkins University Press.

Cassell, E. J. (1985). *Talking with patients* (Vols. 1 & 2). Cambridge, MA: MIT Press.

Dowd, S. B., Poole, V. L., Davidhizar, R., & Giger, J. N. (1998). Death, dying and grief in a transcultural context: Application of the Giger and Davidhizar assessment model. *The Hospice Journal, 13(4)*, 33–56.

Ersek, M., Kagawa-Singer, M., Barnes, D., Blackhall, L., & Koenig, B. A. (1998). Multicultural considerations in the use of advance directives. *Oncology Nursing Forum, 25,* 1683–1690.

Ferszt, G. G., & Houck, P. D. (1986). The family. In M. O. Amenta & N. L. Bohnet (Eds.), *Nursing care of the terminally ill.* Boston: Little, Brown.

Irish, D. P., Lundquist, K. F., & Nelson, V. J. (1993). *Ethnic variations in dying, death, and grief: Diversity in universality.* Washington, DC: Taylor and Francis.

Kagawa-Singer, M. (1998). The cultural context of death rituals and mourning practices. *Oncology Nursing Forum, 25,* 1752–1756.

Kaye, P. (1990). *Notes on symptom control in hospice and palliative care.* Essex, CT: Hospice Education Institute.

Kemp, C. (1995). *Terminal illness: A guide to nursing care.* Philadelphia: Lippincott.

Kübler-Ross, E. (1969). *On death and dying: What the dying have to teach doctors, nurses, clergy, and their own families.* New York: Macmillan.

Lair, G. S. (1996). *Counseling the terminally ill: Sharing the journey.* Bristol, PA: Taylor and Francis.

Larson, D. G. (1993). *The helper's journey: Working with people facing grief, loss, and life-threatening illness.* Champaign, IL: Research Press.

Long, L. (1992). *Understanding/responding: A communication manual for nurses* (2nd ed.). Boston: Jones and Bartlett.

Lugton, J. (1988). *Communicating with dying people and their relatives.* Reading, Berks (England): Austen Cornish Publishers.

Martinson, I. M. (1998). Funeral rituals in Taiwan and Korea. *Oncology Nursing Forum, 25,* 1756–1760.

Monroe, B. (1998). Social work in palliative care. In D. Doyle, G. W. C. Hanks, & N. MacDonald (Eds.), *Oxford textbook of palliative medicine* (2nd ed.). New York: Oxford University Press.

Munet-Vilaro, F. (1998). Grieving and death rituals of Latinos. *Oncology Nursing Forum, 25,* 1761–1763.

Neuberger, J. (1998). Cultural issues in palliative care. In D. Doyle, G. W. C. Hanks, & N. MacDonald (Eds.), *Oxford textbook of palliative medicine* (2nd ed.). New York: Oxford University Press.

Parry, J. K. (1990). *Social work practice with the terminally ill: A transcultural prospective.* Springfield, IL: Charles C Thomas.

Ray, M. C. (1992). *I'm here to help: A hospice worker's guide to communicating with dying people and their loved ones.* Mound, MN: McRay Company.

Rosner, F. (1993). Hospice, medical ethics and Jewish customs. *American Journal of Hospice and Palliative Care, 10(4)*, 6–10.

Weisman, A. D. (1984). *The coping capacity: On the nature of being mortal.* New York: Human Sciences Press.

# CHAPTER 4

# Disease Processes Common to Hospice

**PURPOSE**

The purpose of this chapter is to describe major disease processes likely to result in hospice admission and to introduce potential criteria for shifting from acute care to hospice care.

**OBJECTIVES**

After completing this chapter, the learner will be able to:

1. Write a general definition of end-stage disease, including processes that likely have preceded hospice admission

2. Discuss distressing symptoms or dysfunctions to be anticipated with end-stage disease

3. Name at least two parameters that may signal appropriateness for hospice admission in cancer, cardiac failure, and pulmonary failure

**CONTENT OUTLINE**

   C.  HIV-AIDS

   D.  Pulmonary failure

   E.  Liver failure

   F.  Neurological disorders

   G.  Renal failure

# INTRODUCTION

In the initial development of the modern hospice movement, the focus was solely on patients in the terminal phases of cancer. This was not so much a choice as a response to the large number of patients with end-stage cancer whose pain and other distressing symptoms were being ignored. End-stage cancer remains the predominant diagnosis among patients referred to hospice (about 80%). Heart-related diagnoses account for 10%, and the remaining 10% includes AIDS, renal failure, neurological diseases, and others (Berry, Zeri, & Egan, 1997). This chapter will consider the disease processes that commonly require palliative care and describe some of the parameters for establishing limited prognosis.

Providing good symptom management and improving quality of life for patients with a terminal condition require an understanding of the terminal disease process. An understanding of the pathophysiology of the disease, what treatments the patient has undergone, and likely distressing side effects of the disease and treatments will increase the effectiveness of comfort therapies. Knowledge of the etiology of a particular symptom, whether it be pain or edema, is helpful in determining the most effective intervention. This awareness also prepares us for the kind of patient/family teaching that may strengthen their coping mechanisms.

The usual indications of advanced, progressive, irreversible disease are increasing complications, lack of response to therapies with potential for curing or controlling the disease, more frequent hospitalizations, more intensive care regimens, and decline in the patient's quality of life. Aspects of quality of life include self-care, independence, ability to communicate with the surrounding world, and ability to be involved in activities that bring enjoyment.

# PERFORMANCE STATUS

Regardless of diagnosis, performance status is a common gross measurement of disease progression. Performance status has been included as a variable in cancer research and is one of the factors considered by oncologists in determining potential outcomes of chemotherapy regimens. Performance status is also used to determine prognosis. The Karnofsky Performance Status Scale and the the ECOG (Eastern Cooperative Oncology Group) Scale—also known as the Zubrod Scale—are two scales commonly used to measure performance status (Forster & Lynn, 1989; Reuben, Mor, & Hiris, 1988; Enck, 1990). Table 4.1 lists the parameters of these two scales.

# LIMITED PROGNOSIS CRITERIA

## Estimating Prognosis

General guidelines are available to assist in judging when a patient has a limited prognosis and therefore is an appropriate candidate for hospice referral. Knowledge about estimating prognoses comes from studies of specific diseases (especially cancer) as well as from general critical care studies. In 1976 and continuing through the 1980s, critical care physicians conducted extensive research to develop the APACHE (Acute Physiology and Chronic Health Evaluation), a scoring system for assessing severity of illness, which they correlated to probability of mortality. Though this scoring system did not change critical care practices very much, it did create interest in measurable parameters and predictability of death.

In a study of over 5,000 admissions to intensive care units in thirteen different hospitals, Knaus and colleagues (Knaus, Draper, Wagner, & Zimmerman, 1986; Knaus, Draper, Wagner, & Zimmerman, 1985) found high death rates associated with acute organ system failure (OSF), with rates increasing with number of OSFs and days of duration. The mortality rate of patients with a single OSF lasting more than 1 day was nearly 40%. Two OSFs lasting more than 1 day increased death rates to 60%. Mortality rate for patients with three or more OSFs persisting over 3 days was 98%. Another interesting result of numerous studies is the high correlation between low Karnofsky scores (poor performance status) and short survival times.

The second edition of *Medical Guidelines for Determining Prognosis in Selected Non-Cancer Diseases*, published by the National Hospice Organization (NHO) in 1996, lists over 200 studies of disease states and prognosis. Surprisingly, many of these studies have been for neurological diseases such as amyotrophic lateral sclerosis (ALS) and Alzheimer's, which we might think would be more difficult to measure. Several scales have been developed as staging guidelines for severity of dementia, and studies have been undertaken to check correlation of stage to survival. The limited prognosis guidelines used in this chapter are summarized from the information in the NHO publication; more detail and convenient screening worksheets can be found in that monograph.

## Table 4.1    Parameters of Two Performance Status Scales

| KARNOFSKY | ECOG (OR ZUBROD) |
|---|---|
| 100% Normal, no complaints, no disease | 0 = Fully active; able to carry out predisease activities |
| 90% Able to carry on normal activities; minor signs or symptoms of disease | 1 = Restricted in physically strenuous activity, but ambulatory and able to do light work |
| 80% Normal activities conducted with effort; some symptoms of disease | 2 = Ambulatory and capable of all self-care, but unable to work; up and about more than 50% of waking hours |
| 70% Cares for self; unable to perform normal activity or do active work | |
| 60% Requires occasional assistance, but able to care for most of personal needs | 3 = Capable of limited self-care, confined to bed or wheelchair more than 50% of waking hours |
| 50% Requires considerable assistance and frequent medical care | |
| 40% Disabled; requires special care and assistance | 4 = Completely disabled; no self-care, totally confined to bed or chair |
| 30% Severely disabled; may be hospitalized, death not imminent | |
| 20% Seriously ill; probably in hospital, intensive therapies needed | |
| 10% Moribund; fatal disease progressing rapidly | |
| 0% Dead | |

## General Guidelines for Determining Limited Prognosis

In addition to disease-specific parameters, general guidelines exist for determining limited prognosis regardless of diagnosis. These general guidelines may be summarized as follows:

- A life-limiting condition or disease with either documented clinical progression or recent declining nutritional status related to the terminal condition

- Clinical progression of the disease documented by serial physicals, lab tests, other studies; multiple emergency room visits or hospitalizations; or recent functional status decline, documented by Karnofsky Performance Status of 50% or less or dependence in at least three activities of daily living (e.g., bathing, dressing, feeding, transfers, elimination, or independent ambulation to the bathroom)

◆ Recent decline in nutritional status, documented as unintentional progressive weight loss of greater than 10% over prior 6 months, or albumin less than 2.5 g/dl

These general guidelines (as well as the following disease-specific criteria) should be viewed as *potential criteria* because there is still some debate about whether they are too proscriptive—or even accurate. The authors of the NHO monograph clearly state that the studies they refer to indicate an "increased likelihood of death" and were not done with the specific outcome of 6 months or less in mind. However, some health plans see the guidelines as a protection against abuse of the hospice benefit and are requiring that these criteria be met before admitting a patient to hospice. The challenge is to accept the need for guidelines but to recognize the need for leeway in individual patient differences and physician judgment.

# Specific Disease Processes

# Cancer

## Disease Process

- Leading cancer deaths: lung, colorectal, breast, prostate
- Metastasis leading to organ failure, complications, and death:

    Most common metastatic sites: lymph nodes, lung, bone, and liver

    Most common cancers metastasizing to bone: breast, lung, prostate

    Most common cancers metastasizing to lung: all except bladder, brain, uterus

    Most common cancers metastasizing to brain: breast, kidney, lung, melanoma

- Mechanisms of metastasis:

    Dissemination through lymph system

    Dissemination through circulatory system

    Seeding of a body cavity (i.e., peritoneal)

- Chemotherapy side effects (SE), mostly systemic and reversible:

    SE that subside a few days after treatment but are the most distressing to the patient: nausea, vomiting, diarrhea, anorexia, stomatitis

    SE that subside days to weeks after treatment: neutropenia (patient at high risk of infection)

    SE that may be permanent/chronic: neuropathies (vincristine, vinblastine), nephrotoxicity (cisplatin), cardiotoxicity (doxorubicin), hemorrhagic cystitis (cyclophosphamide), or pancytopenia (if extensive and repeated courses of chemotherapy have been given)

- Radiation (XRT) side effects, totally dependent on dose and site of XRT (damage irreversible):

    Lower abdomen XRT, resulting in chronic cystitis and/or diarrhea

Nerve plexuses XRT, resulting in chronic neuritic pain

Hair loss (only if a full dose has been delivered to the head)

*NOTE:* Low-dose XRT is effective for bone pain and rarely has any side effects.

- Complications of end-stage cancer:

    Cachexia

    Hypercalcemia (most common oncologic emergency)

    Pericardial tamponade (from tumor, metastases, XRT, chemotherapy)

    Bowel obstruction

    Pleural effusion

    Hypercoaguable states (disseminated intravascular coagulation, uncontrolled bleeding and thrombus formation)

    Serum viscosity syndrome (especially with myelomas)

    Spinal cord compression (important to recognize early signs and symptoms)

    Superior vena cava syndrome

    Hemorrhage

    Tumor lysis syndrome (from cell lysis releasing uric acid and intracellular minerals)

## Limited Prognosis Criteria

- Disease progression by local extension or distant metastases despite cancer therapies (no longer responding)

- Declining performance status due to muscle wasting, loss of strength, or pain

- Limited prognosis documented by standard cancer data

- Anorexia with unintentional weight loss and cachexia, with or without nutritional supplementation

- Persistent and increasing intensities of pain

- Multiple disease-related symptoms or complications requiring comfort interventions

# Heart Failure

## Disease Process

- Two major causes of heart failure:

    Cardiomyopathies, with multiple etiologies resulting in degeneration, hypertrophy, or infiltration of myocardium

    Coronary artery disease (CAD) or ischemic heart disease resulting in myocardial infarction or ischemia from insufficient circulation. Risk factors: smoking, hypertension, high cholesterol, stress, obesity

- Treatment for angina and hypertension: vasodilators, diuretics, and beta blockers

- Treatment for improving contractility: digitalis preparations. Signs of digitalis toxicity: abdominal pain, nausea and vomiting, visual problems, bradycardia, anorexia, arrhythmias, headaches, seizures

- Treatment for CAD or cardiomyopathies: ACE (angiotensin-converting enzyme) inhibitors and calcium channel blockers to reduce afterload

- Congestive heart failure activation of the renin-angiotensin-aldosterone system, resulting in sodium retention, which causes fluid retention

- Progressive right-sided failure, affecting the body systemically and resulting in increased dependent peripheral edema and poor perfusion of tissues

- Progressive left-sided failure, resulting in an increase in lung congestion symptoms such as dyspnea, cough, and tachycardia

## Limited Prognosis Criteria

- Inability to carry out any physical activity without discomfort

- Symptoms of heart failure or angina, even at rest

- Ejection fraction of 20% or less

- Persistent symptoms despite optimal treatment with diuretics and vasodilators (treatment failure)

♦ Presence or history of events that further decrease chance of recovery or survival: cardiac arrest, unexplained syncope, cardiogenic brain embolism, AIDS, or symptomatic supraventricular or ventricular arrhythmias that are resistant to antiarrhythmic therapy

# HIV-AIDS

## Disease Process

*NOTE:* Routine care of a patient with AIDS does not require gloves or any kind of isolation; gloves should be worn when handling any body fluids.

♦ HIV virus transmitted via blood, sexual contact, breast milk of HIV-positive mothers

♦ Disease of T-lymphocytes with an affinity for CD4 cells:

> HIV positive and CD4 T-cell count greater than 500, usually asymptomatic

> HIV positive and CD4 T-cell count less than 200, susceptible to life-threatening infections

♦ Early symptoms: thrush, candida or other infections, fever, weight loss, diarrhea

♦ Leading cause of death in HIV-AIDS: opportunistic infections secondary to immunodeficiency

♦ Treatment for HIV with antiretrovirals:

> Zivovudine (AZT, Retrovir, ZDV). Side effects (SE): pancytopenia, nausea and vomiting, diarrhea, dizziness, headache

> Didanosine (ddI, Videx). SE: pancreatitis, neuropathies, seizures, pancytopenia, central nervous system depression

> Zalcitabine (ddc, HIVID). SE: neuropathies, rash, pruritis, fatigue

♦ Treatment for *Pneumocystis carinii* pneumonia (PCP), a major AIDS-defining diagnosis and cause of death:

> Trimethoprim-sulfamethoxazole (TMP-SMX, Bactrim, Septra) as first-line treatment

> If no response or frequent recurrences, add dapsone (DDS, Aviosulfon) or pentamidine

- Treatment for tuberculosis (an aggressive and resistant strain): isoniazid (INH), ethambutol (Myambutol), rifampin (Rifadin), pyrazinamide (Tebrazid), and rifapentine (Priftin)

- Treatment for *Mycobacterium avium* (MAC): rifabutin (Mycobutin). SE: red-orange urine, feces, sputum, sweat and tears; soft contact lenses will be stained

- Treatment for *Cytomegalovirus* (CMV): ganciclovir (Cytovene)

    *NOTE:* CMV can infect brain, organs, gastrointestinal tract, other. A disturbing and disabling symptom for patients is retinitis, accompanied by progressive blindness.

- End-stage complications: wasting syndrome, dementia, infections, and cancer (most commonly Kaposi's sarcoma and lymphomas)

## Limited Prognosis Criteria

*NOTE:* Prognosis may change quickly with development of new drugs.

- Rapid progression of opportunistic infections, persistent wasting, or cancers

- Advanced AIDS dementia

- CD4 T-cell count less than 25 cells/mcL in absence of acute illness

- Viral load (HIV RNA) greater than 100,000 copies/ml

- Viral load (HIV RNA) less than 100,000 copies/ml but with declining functional status, cessation of antiretroviral and prophylactic medications, or presence of complications such as chronic, persistent diarrhea for 1 year; persistent serum albumin less than 2.5 g/dl; continuing substance abuse; age greater than 50 years; or symptomatic congestive heart failure at rest

# Pulmonary Failure

## Disease Process

- Chronic obstructive pulmonary disease (COPD):

    Emphysema type: "pink puffer," barrel-chested, thin, uses accessory muscles to breathe

    Chronic bronchitis type: "blue bloater," overweight, wheezes

- Restrictive lung disease (RLD): decreased vital capacity caused by myasthenia gravis, fibrosis, tumor, effusions, other

- Treatment for COPD: aminophyllin, steroids, inhalers

- Treatment for RLD: steroids, oxygen if not obstructive

- End-stage complications: cor pulmonale (right heart) and respiratory failure; severe dyspnea, which limits activities and elicits fear and anxiety

## Limited Prognosis Criteria

- Disabling dyspnea at rest, accompanied by fatigue, cough and decreased functional activity

- Forced expiratory volume ($FEV_1$) less than 30% of normal predicted value

- Progressive disease documented by increasing emergency room visits or hospitalizations for respiratory failure or pulmonary infections, decrease in $FEV_1$ greater than 40 ml in 1 year

- Cor pulmonale (right heart failure) secondary to pulmonary disease

- Hypoxia (pulmonary oxygen less than 55 mmHg or oxygen saturation less than 88%) at rest and on oxygen administration

- Pulmonary carbon dioxide greater than 50 mmHg

- Unintentional progressive weight loss greater than 10% over past 6 months

- Resting tachycardia greater than 100 beats per minute in patient with known COPD

# Liver Failure

## Disease Process

- Commonly occurs with alcoholic liver cirrhosis or chronic hepatitis caused by viruses, medications, other

- Treatment: usually intensive care for acute episodes and comfort measures

- Disease progression: esophageal varices with risk of hemorrhage, blood dyscrasias, ascites, peritonitis, and dyspnea

## Limited Prognosis Criteria

*NOTE:* In liver disease, clinical judgment is the deciding factor because dramatic improvements are common even in severely decompensated patients.

- Pertinent factors: recurrent episodes of critical liver failure; progression to severely impaired liver function (prothrombin time greater than 5 seconds over control and serum albumin less than 2.5 g/dl); and complications such as refractory ascites, spontaneous bacterial peritonitis, hepatorenal syndrome, refractory hepatic encephalopathy, or recurrent variceal bleeding

- Factors shown to worsen prognosis: progressive malnutrition, muscle wasting with reduced strength and endurance, continued active alcoholism, hepatocellular carcinoma, or hepatitis B surface antigen positivity

# Neurological Disorders

## Disease Process

*NOTE:* For all neurological disorders, disease progression is noted by an increase in injuries from loss of muscle control, body wasting, refractory infections, and a decrease in performance status.

- ◆ Causes of cerebrovascular accident (CVA): plaque, emboli, or aneurysm; widely varying degrees of severity from temporary weakness to death. Treatment: anticoagulants, streptokinase, other

- ◆ Amyotrophic lateral sclerosis (ALS): progressive degeneration of the motor system with no known effective treatment

- ◆ Multiple sclerosis (MS): progressive (usually slow, over many years), random loss of myelin, which results in dysfunction to affected areas because of interrupted nerve conduction. Treatment: mainly supportive care; some use of trials of gamma globulin, corticosteroids, or Interferon ß

- ◆ Alzheimer's disease: usually a diagnosis of exclusion with progressive and irreversible dementia and no known treatment

- ◆ Parkinson's disease: degeneration of the basal ganglia. Treatment: levadopa or benztropine

## Limited Prognosis Criteria

- ◆ Dysphagia severe enough to prevent oral intake in a patient who declines or is not a candidate for artificial nutrition and hydration

- ◆ Poor nutritional status, defined as unintentional progressive weight loss of greater than 10% over prior 6 months, or albumin greater than 2.5 g/dl

- ◆ Medical complications related to declining performance status and progressive clinical decline, such as aspiration pneumonia, pyelonephritis, sepsis, refractory Stage 3 or 4 decubitus ulcers, recurrent fever after antibiotics

- ◆ Coma, with any four of the following on the third day: abnormal brain-stem response, absent verbal response, absent withdrawal response to pain, serum creatinine greater than 1.5 mg/dl, and age greater than 70 years

- Coma or severe obtundance accompanied by severe myoclonus persisting beyond 3 days after anoxic stroke

- End-stage ALS: indicated by widespread muscle deterioration affecting all areas of the body, resulting in impaired ventilatory capacity, life-threatening complications, and critical nutritional impairment (with or without artificial feeding)

- End-stage advanced dementia (from Alzheimer's, multi-infarct, other): patients at least at Stage 7 of the Functional Assessment Staging (FAST; Reisberg, Sclan, Franssen, Kluger, & Ferris, 1994) and showing all of the following—inability to ambulate, bathe, and dress independently; urinary and fecal incontinence; and inability to communicate meaningfully

# Renal Failure

## Disease Process

- Causes: malignancies, toxins, medications, lupus, or diabetes
- May or may not be accompanied by oliguria
- BUN (blood urea nitrogen) and creatinine may rise (azotemia)
- Disease progression: uremia, anemias, fluid/electrolyte imbalance, acid/base imbalances, other

## Limited Prognosis Criteria

- In patients with chronic renal failure, discontinuation of dialysis
- Critical renal failure, defined as creatinine clearance of less than 10 cc per minute and serum creatinine greater than 8 mg/dl
- Any of the following conditions in a patient with renal failure who is not to undergo dialysis: uremia, oliguria, refractory hyperkalemia, uremic pericarditis, hepatorenal syndrome, or intractable fluid overload
- For hospitalized acute renal failure patients, any of the following comorbidities: need for mechanical ventilation, malignancy, chronic lung disease, advanced cardiac disease, advanced liver disease, sepsis, HIV-AIDS or other immunosuppressed states, albumin less than 3.5 g/dl, cachexia, platelet count less than 25,000, age greater than 75 years, disseminated intravascular coagulation, or gastrointestinal bleeding

## REFERENCES AND SUGGESTED READINGS

Berry, P., Zeri, K., & Egan, K. (1997). *The nurse's study guide: A preparation for the CRNH candidate.* Pittsburgh: Hospice and Palliative Nurses Association.

Enck, R. E. (1990). Prognostication of survival in hospice care. *American Journal of Hospice and Palliative Care, 7*(2), 11–13.

Forster, L. E., & Lynn, J. (1989). The use of physiologic measures and demographic variables to predict longevity among inpatient hospice applicants. *American Journal of Hospice Care, 6*(2), 31–34.

Hanrahan, P., & Luchins, D. J. (1995). Feasible criteria for enrolling end-stage dementia patients in home hospice care. *The Hospice Journal, 10*(3), 47–54.

Kinzbrunner, B., & Pratt, M. M. (1994). Severity index scores correlate with survival of AIDS patients. *American Journal of Hospice and Palliative Care, 11*(3), 4–9.

Knaus, W. A., Draper, E. A., Wagner, D. P., & Zimmerman, J. E. (1986). An evaluation of outcome from intensive care in major medical centers. *Annals of Internal Medicine, 104,* 410–418.

Knaus, W. A., Draper, E. A., Wagner, D. P., & Zimmerman, J. E. (1985). Prognosis in acute organ-system failure. *Annals of Surgery, 202*(6), 685–692.

Mor, V., Laliberte, L., Morris, J. N., & Wiemann, M. (1984). The Karnofsky Performance Status Scale: An examination of its reliability and validity in a research setting. *Cancer, 53,* 2002–2007.

National Hospice Organization. (1996). *Medical guidelines for determining prognosis in selected non-cancer diseases* (2nd ed.). Arlington, VA: Author.

Nuland, S. B. (1994). *How we die.* New York: Knopf.

Reisberg, B., Sclan, S. G., Franssen, E., Kluger, A., & Ferris, S. (1994). Dementia staging in chronic care populations. *Alzheimer Disease and Associated Disorders, 8,* S188–S205.

Reuben, D. B., Mor, V., & Hiris, J. (1988). Clinical symptoms and length of survival in patients with terminal cancer. *Archives of Internal Medicine, 148,* 1586–1591.

Volicer, B. J., Hurley, A., Fabiszewski, K. J., Montgomery, P., & Volicer, L. (1993). Predicting short-term survival for patients with advanced Alzheimer's disease. *Journal of the American Geriatric Society, 41*(5), 535–540.

# CHAPTER 5

# Imminent Death

**PURPOSE**

The purpose of this chapter is to describe what may be experienced subjectively by the patient, and those physiological changes that may be observed objectively by caregivers, when the patient is imminently dying.

**OBJECTIVES**

After completing this chapter, the learner will be able to:

1. List some of the physiological changes of approaching death related to skin, circulatory, gastrointestinal, central nervous system, genitourinary, and respiratory systems

2. Relate some examples of near-death experiences a dying patient might report

3. Discuss how these observations relate to anticipatory grief work

**CONTENT OUTLINE**

III. Mental and Spiritual Phenomena

    A.  Mentation

    B.  Social and emotional status

    C.  Spiritual issues

# DYING: A WHOLE-PERSON EXPERIENCE

As the time of death nears, the body goes through a natural process of shutting down. In recent years, with the majority of people dying in hospital settings, we have been somewhat removed from this natural process. Therefore, family and caregivers may feel overwhelmed during this time unless they have emotional support and guidance from the hospice staff. They will need to know that there will be many changes—physical, emotional, spiritual, and mental. From loss of muscle tone to renal failure, the changes are part of the natural process of the body's decline. These phenomena are sometimes referred to as "active dying."

Anticipatory grief work can begin to take place, if it hasn't already, if hospice team members are supportive and point out the signs of the dying process. As family members observe these signs, the certainty of death may become real for the first time. At this point, they may be overwhelmed with thoughts about what it may be like to live without this dying person.

Loved ones also need to know that physical, emotional, mental, and spiritual dimensions may not decline simultaneously. As a result, we see patients who from an emotional standpoint are not "ready to die," but whose bodies can no longer continue to function. Conversely, some patients have accepted their impending deaths and become impatient waiting for their bodies to catch up to their emotions. At other times, we see patients who appear able to control the time of their death, who will themselves to stay alive until a certain thing happens or a certain person comes to visit. There is no explaining this part of our human nature.

Following are some of the points to remember as the patient is nearing the death event:

- ◆ Dying happens to all dimensions of the person—physical, emotional, spiritual, mental.

- ◆ Death is a natural and normal process.

- ◆ All body systems begin to shut down; the failure of one affects the others.

- The spirit (or soul, or life force) begins to release from the body.

- Near-death experiences may occur (e.g., visions or out-of-body phenomena).

- All dimensions of mind and body may not progress simultaneously.

- Interest in surroundings, events, and socialization generally decreases.

- Sleep increases.

- Phenomena may occur abruptly or very slowly.

Comforting interventions when the patient is actively dying include the following:

- Continue to explain your actions.

- Anticipate needs; don't force talking.

- Watch for nonverbal signs of pain (groaning, grimacing, restlessness).

- Remember the value of presence.

- Maintain a calm atmosphere.

- Encourage family members to communicate their feelings.

- Understand that medication may need to be given by new routes; pain does not stop when the patient can no longer verbalize it.

- Show continued respect for the person and the body.

# PHYSICAL CHANGES

## Physical Appearance

The loss of muscle tone and body energy results in many objective physical changes. As Dr. Robert Enck (1994) explains, when hepatic and renal failure occur, the body and brain are unable to cope with hypoxia, malnutrition, electrolyte imbalance, tumor burden, and toxins that are not cleared from the body. These changes will be distressing to family members, and they may need encouragement to be present and to offer comfort to the patient. They need to know that these processes are usual and expected; they also need to be reminded that the patient is usually oblivious to the changes in the late stages of illness.

The following list summarizes expected changes in physical appearance:

- Skin may be pale, blue, or gray.

- Lips and fingernail beds may be very blue.

- Skin may feel cool, unless there is fever.

- Nose and chin may appear pointed.

- Eyes and cheeks may be sunken.

- Earlobes may fall back toward the cranium.

- Eyes may be half-open.

- Neck may hyperextend.

- Lower jaw may relax, and mouth will be open.

- Skin may become more fragile.

- The possibility of bruising will increase, especially with certain conditions (e.g., liver failure, low platelet count, leukemia).

It will be necessary to prepare family members for changes to expect and explain why the changes are occurring. Specific interventions that will be therapeutic for the patient are as follows:

- If the patient's eyes are open, provide artificial tears for moisture.

- Moisturize and cleanse mouth frequently to prevent dryness and crusting.

- Dry skin by gentle patting, not firm rubbing.

- If bleeding potential is present, take extra care with shaving and hold pressure to any injection site for 10 minutes.

## Circulation

When the heart is failing, blood circulation will be slower and pressure will decrease. Organs and body tissues will be poorly perfused and therefore poorly oxygenated. Peripheral circulation declines first as the body conserves the waning functions for vital organs. Eventually, the vital organs also fail.

The following list summarizes expected changes in circulatory function:

- Heart fails in pumping function, resulting in ischemia and/or pulmonary congestion and other fluid retention (e.g., dependent edema and abdominal distention).

- Blood pressure drops.

- Pulse rate accelerates.

- Pulse becomes progressively weaker and more irregular.

- Lack of perfusion may increase wound necrosis.

- Extremities become ashen, cool, and mottled.

- Lips, nail beds, earlobes, and fingers may look bluish.

- Poor kidney perfusion results in decreased output and increased toxins.

In addition to teaching the family about these changes, therapeutic measures for the patient include the following:

- Keep the patient warm, but avoid electric or heavy blankets.

- Provide good wound care.

- Give cool sponge bath and/or acetaminophen if the patient is restless with fever.

## Metabolism

In a terminal state, almost always with multisystems failure, it becomes evident not only that the patient has less interest in eating or drinking but that proper absorption and metabolism do not occur. This means the patient will not benefit from forced feeding or artificially provided feedings. The patient rarely complains of hunger or thirst and is more comfortable in a dehydrated state. Artificially provided nutrition and hydration can produce distressing side effects, such as lung congestion, edema, and nausea. When hospice team members point out the differences in comfort levels and provide printed material on the subject, most family members will confirm these observations.

The following list summarizes changes in metabolism that occur in the dying process:

- The need for food and interest in food decrease.

- The digestive and metabolic functions slow down, resulting in inability to use artificially provided food and fluid.

- Edema results from decreased metabolism, decreased protein intake, decreased activity, and inefficient renal and cardiac function.

- Poor liver and kidney function may result in indigestion, flatus, and diarrhea.

- Nausea is common.

- The abdomen may become distended.

- Hiccups sometimes occur.

- Fever is common near death, resulting from tumor fever (hypermetabolic activity of cancer cells), dehydration, or loss of temperature regulation in the brain.

- Swallowing and gag reflexes disappear.

- Weakness increases.

Because eating and drinking are habits associated with life and caring, there are always strong feelings about the topic. It is helpful to explain the metabolic process to family and significant others, suggest other ways of showing caring, and emphasize what makes the patient more comfortable. Palliative interventions for symptoms resulting from metabolic changes include the following:

- Provide only intake desired and tolerated by the patient.

- Do not force food or fluids.

- Give ice chips or frozen juice pops if they are appealing.

- Clean and lubricate the patient's mouth and lips.

- Remove dentures if desired.

- In the presence of persistent vomiting, check for constipation (depending on disease trajectory).

- Medicate to prevent nausea.

- Seek medication to help hiccups. (Thorazine is useful.)

- Assist desired activity; do not insist on undesired activity.

## Respiration

Changes in respiratory rate, rhythm, and efficiency occur secondary to metabolic imbalance, tumor or fluid prevention of oxygen–carbon dioxide exchange, or exacerbated chronic lung disorders. If the cardiac muscle is also functioning poorly, oxygen perfusion and oxygen–carbon dioxide exchange proceed in a downward spiral of inefficiency. In addition, dyspnea is almost always accompanied by distress and anxiety. Between the anxiety and the pathophysiology, tachypnea and oxygen saturation worsen. So, the therapeutic approach is twofold: utilization of calming measures and administration of medication to relax the lung parenchyma chemically. Both measures will help in slowing inefficient hyperventilation.

Noisy and moist respirations result from fluid retention and lack of either muscle tone or strength to cough up secretions. On rare occasions suctioning may give relief, but generally it does not result in preventing the symptoms, nor does it increase comfort. Cough is common if reflex is still present and if fluid, secretions, or tumor exist anywhere in the respiratory tract.

The following list summarizes expected changes in respiratory system functioning:

- Breathing patterns change: slower, faster, labored, apnea, Cheyne Stokes, other.

- Rales occur due to fluid accumulation in the lungs.

- Hypoxia or hypercarbia may cause confusion, irritability, sense of impending doom, fear, or anxiety.

- "Death rattle," or sound of fluids accumulating in the trachea, will be heard.

- Edema of laryngeal area affects swallowing and may produce sound of stridor.

The following interventions for respiratory distress will increase the patient's comfort:

- Decrease perception of dyspnea with cool cloths, fan, or open window.

- Utilize low-dose morphine to reduce respiratory rate to normal.

- Administer codeine to relieve cough.

- Consider antianxiety agents to address psychological component.

- Use scopalamine to dry secretions.

- Elevate the head of the patient's bed.

- Provide reassuring, calm presence.

- Allow the patient to decide on fluid intake; pushing fluids may increase symptoms.

- Turn the patient's head or position on side to drain secretions.

## Elimination

With decreased intake, inefficient circulation, and kidney failure, the urinary output will become scant and concentrated. Urinary retention and/or frequent bed-wetting can be relieved with an indwelling catheter. If frequent bed-wetting is not distressing to the patient or the caregiver, frequent cleansing and pad changes may be preferred.

Decreasing bowel functions result from decreased stimulation secondary to poor intake, lack of exercise, and medications that decrease motility. Cathartics, enemas, and other usual methods of relieving constipation are carried out depending on the condition of the patient and the trajectory of dying. If death is imminent and the patient experiences pain or dyspnea on movement or exertion, then it is not in the patient's best interest to initiate treatment for constipation. If this problem has been managed well prior to the period of active dying, it is not likely to be a prominent symptom.

The following changes in elimination are commonly seen:

- Output of urine and stool decreases.
- Urine becomes more concentrated and darker in color.
- Discomfort results from urinary retention.
- Incontinence is common.

Interventions for elimination problems include the following comfort measures:

- Keep the patient dry and clean.
- Catheterize if the patient is in retention or distressed by frequency or incontinence.
- Treat constipation if the patient is distressed and can tolerate the treatment.

## The Senses

When the patient is actively dying—in the last days, hours, or minutes—there will be a cascading decline in interactions, strength, muscle tone, and so forth. As this happens, the senses decline as well: sight, hearing, touch, smell, and taste. It is thought that hearing is the last sense to be lost and, therefore, right up to the time of death, we should presume that the patient hears everything being said. It is important at this time to talk *to* the patient, not *about* him or her. It is also important to convey calm reassurance, caring, and any special messages thought to be important for the patient to know.

The following list summarizes changes in the senses seen near the time of death:

- Vision may become blurred.

- The eyes may become glassy, with a distant look.

- Senses may be overactive or underactive.

- Hearing may become more acute.

- Sensation of pain may be expressed by moaning or restlessness.

- Patient may become agitated or restless, especially if left alone.

It will be important to assure the family that the patient's lack of response is not rejection. Interventions to provide comfort when there are sensory changes are as follows:

- Always assume the dying person can hear.

- Speak directly to the dying person, even when there is no response.

- Touch the patient gently and remain present.

- Provide a calm atmosphere with minimal stimulation.

- Use artificial tears if the patient's eyes are partially open.

## MENTAL AND SPIRITUAL PHENOMENA

### Mentation

There are many reasons mental status changes occur in the dying process, including liver failure, renal failure, decreased oxygenation to the brain, or toxicities from medications. Reassuring calmness and medications to relax the patient will be of benefit. It becomes more important than ever to communicate with the patient and listen patiently to what he or she is saying. It is futile at this point to try to argue about what the patient says or means. Rather, try to understand what the patient is trying to convey to you. It is not a time to make demands on or unrealistic requests of the patient. Especially, this should not be a time to manipulate the patient into decisions to benefit survivors.

The following list summarizes changes in mentation commonly seen in dying patients:

- Level of consciousness may vary widely.

- Fatigue and sleep may increase; coma state may occur.

- Confusion, agitation, or restlessness may be present.

- The patient may do any of the following:

Pick at the air or bed covers

Have muscle twitching in extremities

Say strange things or seem not to make sense

Be disoriented as to time and place

Be confused about familiar people

The following interventions may provide comfort to patients experiencing a change in mentation:

- Continue to talk to the dying person.

- Assess when restlessness is a sign of pain or other discomfort.

- Offer calm reassurances, gentle massage, or discussion of pleasant memories.

- Medicate for restlessness or agitation.

- Administer muscle relaxants to help reduce muscle twitching.

- Try to make a connection with the patient's words.

- Identify yourself to the patient; do not ask the patient to identify you.

- Explain to the patient what is happening prior to any procedure.

- Provide soothing music or readings if the patient's preferences are known.

- Suggest patient/family/physician discussion of drug-induced sedation if the patient is in extreme distress and symptoms cannot be controlled. (This situation is extremely rare.)

- Avoid restraints unless absolutely necessary for patient safety; if used, always undo restraints when someone can be present with the patient.

## Social and Emotional Status

At the end of life, it is common for the dying person to become more introspective and less interested in what is happening around him or her. Energy or the interest to discuss business affairs or family matters may diminish. For this reason, it is important to address concerns whenever the patient brings them up, preferably at an earlier stage of the terminal diagnosis when the patient still has the capacity to reason and communicate. Ignoring or putting off patient concerns may rob the person of the opportunity to do what is most important.

Even when team members, family, or significant others do open the door to unfinished business, some patients will refuse to take the opportunity to act and will die with unresolved conflicts or problems. In this case, they may not experience a peaceful death. Family or other loved ones and team members need to remind themselves that if the opportunity is offered and the patient refuses to take action, then it is beyond their control or responsibility. Resolution is not something that can be forced.

The following list summarizes commonly seen changes in the social and emotional realm. The patient may:

- Resist dying because of concern for family members
- Wish to complete unfinished business
- Decrease socialization (withdrawal is common)
- Be more upset in the presence of certain people
- Express specific concerns about matters such as finances or house repairs
- Be distressed over loss of control or function

  Hospice team members can help the family in these ways:

- Explain changes and prepare the family for what to expect. (This will help them in their anticipatory grief.)
- Encourage the family to give the patient permission to let go, when appropriate.
- Encourage family members to take the opportunity to talk to the patient even when there is no response; it may be a last opportunity to share something important with the patient.
- Explain to family members and patient that tears need not be suppressed; they are normal and show caring.

Specific interventions to relieve the patient's psychosocial distresses include the following:

- Listen to last wishes or confessions.
- Be aware and respect the fact that an occasional patient will wish to be alone.
- Communicate to the patient that what is happening is natural and OK.

## Spiritual Issues

When a person is near death, he or she may experience visions of deceased relatives, Jesus, God, or the like. Although hallucinations or drug reactions are always a possibility, this is not the only explanation: Experiences like these are not uncommon at the end of life. It would be inappropriate to explain away, deride, or deny any experiences patients report. It is far better to let patients share what they are experiencing without any explanation or interpretation. They need to know someone is with them and be assured that these experiences are normal, especially if they seem afraid. The last hours are an opportunity to comfort and honor patients as people, letting them remain in control to whatever degree possible.

The following list summarizes changes commonly seen in the spiritual realm when death is near. The patient may:

- Experience a dream or vision of someone who has already died
- Talk about taking a trip or a journey
- Use phrases like "going home" or "catching the train"
- Talk about bright lights, peace, Jesus, or God
- Remove clothing
- Be fearful of unknown, unfinished business
- Be sad at leaving loved ones behind
- Express a need to forgive or be forgiven by specific individuals
- Request confession or other rituals
- "Choose" time of death (e.g., wait for the arrival of a particular person)
- Express definite wishes about funeral or memorial service

It will be important to encourage the family to forgive, ask forgiveness, and give the patient permission to die, when appropriate. The following specific interventions are comforting for patients in spiritual distress:

- Allow and encourage patient to share experiences.
- Do not restrain the patient or insist on different behavior.
- Listen for meaning or meaningful experience.
- Be present in case the patient wishes to "right" things.
- Do not impose your beliefs or interpretations.
- Be willing to pray, read scriptures, or play music if the patient desires.

## REFERENCES AND SUGGESTED READINGS

Enck, R. E. (1994). The final moments. In R. E. Enck (Ed.), *The medical care of terminally ill patients*. Baltimore: Johns Hopkins University Press.

Kaye, P. (1989). *Notes on symptom control in hospice and palliative care*. Essex, CT: Hospice Education Institute.

Kemp, C. (1995). Imminent death and interventions. In C. Kemp (Ed.), *Terminal illness: A guide to nursing care*. Philadelphia: Lippincott.

Nuland, S. B. (1994). *How we die*. New York: Knopf.

Smith, S. A. (1997). Controversies in hydrating the terminally ill patient. *Journal of Intravenous Nursing, 20*(4), 193–200.

Twycross, R. G., & Lichter, I. (1993). The terminal phase. In D. Doyle, G. W. C. Hanks, & N. MacDonald (Eds.), *Oxford textbook of palliative medicine*. New York: Oxford University Press.

Volker, B. G., Berry, P. H., Egan, K., Eighmy, J. B., Kalina, K., Gallagher-Allred, C. R., Murphy, P. L., Nahman, E. J., Rooney, E. C., Smith, S. A., & Zeri, K. (1999). *Hospice and palliative nursing practice review* (3rd ed.). Pittsburgh: Hospice and Palliative Nurses Association.

Vullo-Navich, K., Smith, S., Andrews, M., Levine, A. M., Tischler, J. F., & Veglia, J. M. (1998). Comfort and incidence of abnormal serum sodium, BUN, creatinine and osmolality in dehydration of terminal illness. *American Journal of Hospice and Palliative Care, 15*(2), 77–84.

Zerwekh, J. (1991). Supportive care of the dying patient. In S. B. Baird, R. McCorkle, & M. Grant (Eds.), *Cancer nursing: A comprehensive textbook*. Philadelphia: W. B. Saunders.

# CHAPTER 6

# Concepts of Grief and Bereavement

**PURPOSE**

The purpose of this chapter is to review well-known theories concerning the grief of dying patients, grief experienced by survivors, and therapeutic approaches to facilitate the bereavement process

**OBJECTIVES**

Upon completion of this chapter, the learner will be able to:

1. Define the five stages of death and dying as identified by Elisabeth Kübler-Ross

2. Identify three of the fears related to death and dying

3. Identify four of the loss issues for dying patients and their families

4. List the four stages of grief resolution according to J. William Worden

5. Discuss therapeutic approaches to bereaved persons

**CONTENT OUTLINE**

I. Theories and Definitions

   A.  Stages of dying

   B.  Emotional components (losses, fears, hope)

   C.  Meaningful tasks of dying patients

II. Grief Process

   A.  Assessing grief needs

# THEORIES AND DEFINITIONS

## Stages of Dying

Dr. Elisabeth Kübler-Ross, in her landmark work on the experiences of dying patients, identified five common reactions: denial, anger, bargaining, depression, and acceptance. She called these the "stages of dying" (see Table 6.1). Some debate that these stages hold true or are applicable to hospice work. However, as reactions they are indeed commonly experienced and applicable to any dying person. Important points to remember are that not every individual will experience all five stages and that the stages do not necessarily represent sequential steps. Any of the reactions can coexist or be revisited many times.

Through the work of Harvard professor Dr. J. William Worden, clinical psychologist Dr. Therese A. Rando, and others, we have broadened our concepts of the dying experience. The following definitions form the basis of our understanding.

- *Grief* is the process of psychological, social, and somatic reactions to perceived loss. The emotional feelings of anger, frustration, guilt, loneliness, and so on are expected and natural reactions to loss. Grief applies to any loss (e.g., divorce, job, self-esteem), but death is generally viewed as the ultimate loss, a universal experience of loss encountered repeatedly throughout life.

- *Anticipatory grief* begins when one becomes aware of a terminal condition (a future loss). The time between knowing death is inevitable and the actual death event offers the opportunity to resolve conflicts or finish business. Hospice staff can prepare the patient, family, and friends for what to expect at the time of death and let them know it is OK to begin to prepare for life after the death.

## Table 6.1 Kübler-Ross's Stages of Death and Dying

**DENIAL**

Disbelief that event could be true

Creation of alternative explanations

Functions as a buffer after unexpected shocking news

**ANGER**

Reaction of rage, envy, resentment, or "Why me?"

Usually displaced at random: doctors, nurses, family, God, and so forth

Results in outbursts and unreasonable demands

**BARGAINING**

An attempt to postpone the inevitable

Mostly with God; promises of good behavior

Promises sometimes associated with quiet guilt

**DEPRESSION**

A normal reaction to realization of great loss

Necessary to experience and express sorrow to facilitate the state of acceptance

Not to be ignored or reasoned away

**ACCEPTANCE**

More void of feeling than "happy"

Circle of interest diminishes

Sitting in silence may be most meaningful communication

---

+ *Mourning* is the cultural reaction to or outward social expression of the loss. It is the way in which one who has suffered a loss adapts from what was to what is. It is a journey of searching and yearning.

+ *Bereavement* is the state of deprivation following the loss of something held to be significant, whether positive or negative.

## Emotional Components

### Losses

Loss, the source of grief, can come in many different forms. The patient who has a terminal illness with progressive complications has the potential for enormous losses. Consciously or subconsciously, the patient will be grieving from current losses, anticipated future losses, and compounded losses from the past. The following list includes some of the possible losses experienced by a dying patient:

- Loss of control and independence
- Loss of future existence and dreams and hopes for the future
- Loss of meaning and aspects of the self and identity
- Loss of significant others
- Loss of familiar environment and possessions

### Fears

Fears are variable, but the three most commonly reported by dying patients are as follows:

- Fear of unrelieved pain
- Fear of abandonment or being alone
- Fear of powerlessness/helplessness

Fear of death itself is further down the list and usually involves fear of the unknown. All human beings experience some degree of fear when faced with an unknown, unfamiliar, and unpredictable event. Hospice staff can help with questions such as "What will happen to my body after death?" Fears about fate in the hereafter may need to be referred to clergy. Whatever the fears, and whether or not we have answers, patients need to know it is safe for them to express what they are thinking.

### Hope

Hope, according to Kübler-Ross, persists despite all the losses, all the fears, and all the grief. The first challenge to all members of the hospice team is to discard the traditional medical meaning of hope, that hope is for a cure alone. Rather, we need a new insight, that there can be many different kinds of hope, even after a patient has been told that there is nothing else that can be done to reverse the disease. The hospice view is that there is much that can be done and many hopes that can be fulfilled.

There is a difference between giving up hope and giving up a particular hope. Dying patients may need some guidance to transfer or realign their hopes. For example, if you ask a patient, "What are your goals?" and the patient responds, "To get well," the next question could be, "And if that can't happen, then what would your goals be?" Hope can be transferred from medical technology to high-level caring. Patients may have hope that they will not be abandoned, hope that they will be free of pain, or hope that others will carry on their work and values. Hope can be thought of in the following ways:

- True hope is always based in reality.
- Hope can and does change as one's reality changes.
- Finding areas of control in a threatening situation enhances hope.
- Each person's hope is personal and unique.
- Hope seems to follow a progressive path of development.

## Meaningful Tasks of Dying Patients

At a symposium at the Connecticut Hospice in 1979, syndicated columnist Jory Graham spoke to the audience about what it was like to be a cancer patient. She was in the process of writing a book about understanding the human needs of cancer patients. Published in 1982, the book was entitled *In the Company of Others: Understanding the Human Needs of Cancer Patients*. But what she said that day was that she planned to call it *The Need to Leave a Mark*. She said she had learned from personal experience and from other patients that the most important thing at the end of life was to know that life had meaning and had served a purpose. She then talked about some of the ways in which this knowledge could be realized.

In the intervening years, much has been written by patients and clinicians about what activities might be most meaningful in one's last days. In emphasizing his belief that the last days represent an opportunity for personal growth, hospice doctor Ira Byock (1996) summarized these activities (see Table 6.2).

Because in their lives many people fail to reach the ultimate goal of self-actualization, as conceived by Maslow (1954), we cannot assume that patients will have interest in relationships and meaning in their last days. Some patients will be too ill or lack the physical or emotional energy to deal with any of these issues. The hospice perspective should be one of recognizing the tasks as having potential for inner healing if the patient chooses to pursue them. Hospice staff can make a difference by being open to inner agony when it exists and by supporting the ways patients choose to deal with it.

# GRIEF PROCESS

## Assessing Grief Needs

A grief assessment is usually done fairly soon after the patient's admission to hospice. Because some of the same information requested to determine care needs will be pertinent to grief needs, this type of assessment is sometimes done in connection with the evaluation of care needs. Ideally, grief assessment occurs early enough that

## Table 6.2   Byock's Tasks of Dying Patients

DEVELOP A RENEWED SENSE OF PERSONHOOD AND MEANING

Find meanings in life through life review and personal narrative

Develop a sense of worthiness, both in the past and in the current situation

Learn to accept love and caring from other people

BRING CLOSURE TO PERSONAL AND COMMUNITY RELATIONSHIPS

Say good-bye to family members and friends with expressions of regret, gratitude, appreciation, and affection

Ask for and grant forgiveness to estranged friends and family members so reconciliation can occur

Say good-bye to community relationships (employment, civic and religious organizations) with expressions of regret, gratitude, forgiveness, and appreciation

BRING CLOSURE TO WORLDLY AFFAIRS

Arrange for the transfer of fiscal, legal, and social responsibilities

Accept the finality of life and surrender to the transcendent

Express the depth of personal tragedy that dying may represent and acknowledge the totality of personal loss

Withdraw from the world and accept increased dependency

Develop a sense of awe and accept the seeming chaos that can prefigure transcendence

---

there can be a plan for anticipatory grief work and so those at risk for complicated bereavement reactions can be identified.

A general assessment will probably cover relationships, coping abilities, support systems, spiritual/religious beliefs, and other life stressors. For grief needs, it would be important to add history of previous responses to losses and degree of preparedness for the patient's death. It is a good idea to have a specific method of assessing grief needs, followed by a plan of care extending into the bereavement period.

A variety of assessment scales in the literature are specific to grief needs. The Holmes and Rahe Social Readjustment Scale (Holmes & Rahe, 1967) has also been employed to identify individuals at risk due to high stress levels. Sometimes a few simple questions can be less threatening to the family member and get at the needed information more quickly than formal assessment. A sample grief assessment questionnaire shown in Table 6.3 lists pertinent questions.

## Table 6.3   Sample Grief Assessment

Anticipating the death of a loved one can be very difficult and stressful. Any of the following information that you care to share with the hospice team will assist us in being more supportive to you. All information is confidential and is for use of the hospice staff only.

1. Are you currently receiving medical care, mental health counseling, or pastoral counseling?
2. What previous losses have you had (i.e., mother, father, brother, sister), and how have you coped?
3. How will the death of _____ change your life?
4. What is your current emotional support system?
5. How do you usually handle stress in your life?
6. How would you describe your relationship with _____?
7. Have you been able to talk openly about matters that need to be taken care of at the time of, and following, _____'s death?
8. How do you feel the hospice staff can be helpful to you?

## Physical, Emotional, and Cognitive Responses to Grief

During bereavement, there will be a series of reactions, both internal and external, to the loss of a close relationship. There is no right way to grieve, nor one right length of time for grieving. Work with the bereaved must include an educational component to prepare them for the grief process and to help them understand what constitutes normal grieving. Many bereaved persons may be frightened by what they experience emotionally and may feel they are "going crazy." They need to be assured that these physical, emotional, and cognitive phenomena can be expected among those who have suffered a loss. These common responses to grief are listed in Table 6.4.

## Tasks or Stages of Grief Resolution

Grief and mourning are very individual experiences, depending on cultural background, spiritual beliefs, previous life experiences, and usual coping patterns. Therefore, we cannot predict time frames or patterns of progression for any specific person. The tasks of grief resolution are not progressive. For example, it is not abnormal for one to be working on reinvesting emotional energy in another relationship and suddenly have the need to relive the loss.

## Table 6.4   Common Responses to Grief

| PHYSICAL | EMOTIONAL | COGNITIVE |
| --- | --- | --- |
| Insomnia | Emotional outbursts | Poor concentration |
| Chest tightness | Frequent crying | Preoccupation with thoughts of the deceased |
| Dry mouth | Irritability | |
| Fatigue | Anxiety | |
| Loss of sexual interest | Hostile reactions/anger | Dreams of the deceased |
| Appetite changes | Overactivity to avoid feelings of guilt | Sense of presence of the deceased |
| Palpitations | | |
| Breathlessness | Loneliness | Visual and auditory hallucinations |
| Decreased energy and strength | Helplessness | Confusion |
| Gastrointestinal disturbances | Lack of feeling/numbness | Disbelief |
| Throat tension | Sense of depersonalization | Idealization (repression of negative thoughts) |
| Susceptibility to illness | Social withdrawal | |
| Restlessness | Depression/sadness | |

From the research and experience of clinicians specializing in care of people in grief, common patterns of grief reactions and grief resolution emerge. Table 6.5 illustrates some of these similarities and relationships. The early work of Parkes (e.g., Parkes, 1970) described the mourning process from the perspective of what the griever experiences. His later work with Weiss (e.g., Parkes & Weiss, 1983) identified phases of grief recovery. Worden (1991) identified four tasks of mourning, the term *task* suggesting goals and implying that there is something mourners can do in this life circumstance. This view in no way negates the intensity and necessity of normal grief reactions; however, it does redirect focus on the process of resolution. Rando (1984, 1993, 2000) looks at the progress of grief resolution in terms of six "R" processes of mourning. She points out that, although various theorists use different labels, they cover the same basic feelings.

Exploring Worden's four tasks of mourning provides insight into the experiences of each phase, which in turn guides us in deciding which approaches will be most therapeutic. Worden also reminds us that grief work is strenuous and draining, and that most people must take it in small segments. Uninterrupted intensity would be over-

## Table 6.5 Tasks or Stages of Grief Resolution

| PARKES' PHASES OF MOURNING | PARKES AND WEISS'S TASKS FOR GRIEF RECOVERY | RANDO'S SIX "R" PROCESSES OF MOURNING | WORDEN'S FOUR TASKS OF MOURNING |
|---|---|---|---|
| Numbness, shock, and disbelief | Intellectual recognition and explanation of loss | Recognize the loss | To accept the reality of the loss |
| Pining, yearning, searching, protest | Emotional acceptance of the loss | React to the separation | To experience the pain of grief |
| Disorganization, despair, depression | Assumption of a new identity | Recollect and reexperience the deceased/lost object and the relationship | To adjust to an environment in which the deceased is missing |
| Reorganization, recovery | | Relinquish the old attachments to the deceased/lost object and the old assumptive world | To emotionally relocate the deceased and move on with life |
| | | Readjust to move adaptively into the new world without forgetting the old | |
| | | Reinvest | |

whelming. Thus, we see periodic returns to denial or avoidance as a natural defense mechanism.

### Task I: To Accept the Reality of the Loss

In this phase, the grieving person may be experiencing denial or shock and disbelief. Denial can relate to the actual death, to the meaning of the loss, or to the permanence of the loss. The finality of death seems unreal, and it is difficult to internalize that the loss actually has happened. Accepting the reality of death takes time because it is both an intellectual and an emotional adjustment.

### Task II: To Experience the Pain of Grief

The pain of grief must be experienced in order to proceed to some degree of resolution. The pain can be, and usually is, both physical and emotional. Common ways in which people avoid this pain is by using alcohol or drugs, avoiding reminders of the dead, and avoiding any possible negative or ambivalent feelings by idealizing the deceased. Avoiding conscious grieving can lead to true depression, physical illness, or aberrant behaviors. In this phase, it is important that people in grief be permitted to express the pain, the agony of soul, anger at the deceased, anger at God, self-pity, and other strong emotions. The hospice professional must be able to hear the sadness the bereaved are feeling and not rush to make them "feel better." Rituals and ceremonies allow grief to be acknowledged in a symbolic and formal way and provide an opportunity for the expression of feelings and personal, spiritual, social, ethnic, and family beliefs.

### Task III: To Adjust to an Environment in Which the Deceased Is Missing

This phase of adjustment involves roles, responsibilities, and a new sense of self. Deterrents to working through this task would be an overwhelming sense of inadequacy or an unhealthy self-identity, a particular possibility if the deceased was a controlling person and/or if the survivor has a dependent personality. The survivor may need to learn new skills, assume new roles, and take on new responsibilities. The changes may be relatively minor, such as learning to drive or take care of the bills. They also may be overwhelming: dealing with living alone, having an empty house, or feeling alone even when people are around. It may take an extended period of time to discover the full impact of the loss and all the accompanying changes, then to feel in control again.

### Task IV: To Emotionally Relocate the Deceased and Move On with Life

Central to this task is understanding that one never forgets the deceased and that the pain never totally goes away. Loss is so difficult for some people that they consciously or subconsciously resolve never to love again. This is probably the most difficult task, but it can be accomplished if one can realize that loving other people is possible without diminishing the love that existed for the deceased.

Volkan (1985) describes this idea in the following way: "A mourner never altogether forgets the dead person who was so highly valued in life and never totally withdraws his investment in his representation. We can never purge those who have been close to us from our own history except by psychic acts damaging to our own identity" (p. 326). The goal is not to stop remembering but to be able to remember with less pain. Shuchter and Zisook (1986) enlarge on the idea of relocating: "A survivor's readiness to enter new relationships depends not on 'giving up' the dead spouse but on finding a suitable place for the spouse in the psychological life of the bereaved—a place that is important but that leaves room for others" (p. 297). Sigmund Freud, cited in E.L. Freud (1961), wrote in a letter to a friend whose son had died that "We find a place for what we lose. Although we know that after such a loss the acute stages of mourning will subside, we also know that we shall remain inconsolable and will never find a substitute. No matter what may fill the gap, even if it be filled completely, it nevertheless remains something else" (p. 386).

Therapeutic clinicians need to be aware that, in one sense, mourning might be considered finished when the griever can emotionally relocate the deceased and reinvest energy in new relationships. At the same time, in the sense that one cannot return to a pregrief state, mourning may never be finished.

## Recognizing Abnormal or Complicated Grief

The people most prone to complicated grief are those who fail to grieve for the present loss and/or have past unresolved losses. Other barriers to grief resolution include guilt, a conflicted premorbid relationship with the deceased, a highly dependent relationship, and poor coping patterns. The last, poor coping patterns, may be from substance abuse, mental illness, poor physical health, or lack of adequate support networks. Sometimes survivors grieve for what they wished for and never had or will never have. If the deceased was an abusive person, the survivor may feel relieved and glad the person is gone. When the survivor does not feel safe in verbalizing these presumably unacceptable emotions, his or her psyche may be overtaxed.

Because bereavement is so individual and variable, there is no specific way to diagnose complicated grief. However, it is important to recognize when a person needs specialized help beyond the expertise of the hospice team. Hospice team members will be on the alert if the assessment has shown some of the high-risk factors mentioned previously. Part of the picture will be an intensification and prolongation of normal grief reactions, which are all-consuming and affect all aspects of the person's life. Other indicators may include the following:

- Severe deterioration of functional status
- Substance abuse
- Morbid preoccupation with worthlessness (loss of self-esteem)
- Self-destructive behaviors or thoughts about suicide
- Minor events triggering major grief reactions
- False euphoria subsequent to the death
- Radical changes in lifestyle
- Exclusion of family, friends, or activities associated with deceased
- Phobias about illness or death

Rando (1993) suggests three variables to consider: absence of a normal grief reaction, prolongation of a normal grief reaction, or distortion of a normal grief reaction. Any one of these responses must then be compared to the full range of normal grief and considered in the context of the specific person's psychological, social, and physiological parameters.

## Issues with Children

It is erroneous to think that children cannot handle death and other losses. Kübler-Ross (1975) says we do them a great disservice when for the sake of protecting them we deprive them of the experience of being around people who are dying. She says those kinds of efforts create unnecessary fear. Children are not born with fears; adults instill fear in them.

There is no need to expose children to agonal suffering or grotesque physical problems, but they do need to experience the reality of death as a natural and expected part of life. Factors that inhibit the mourning process in children include neglect of security needs, poor adult coping models, lack of opportunity to ask questions and express feelings, and ambivalence toward the deceased.

A number of books have been written to explain death to children, and these can be helpful if they fit the family's values and religious beliefs. It is usually sufficient to allow children to be present and to answer their questions honestly. It is important that they not feel neglected nor left alone. Specific approaches depend on the developmental stage of the child and how involved the child wishes to be. Table 6.6 gives a brief summary of children's developmental stages and their concepts of death.

General guidelines for interacting with children when they are experiencing a death include the following:

- Assure children of all ages that they are not at fault.

- Answer questions truthfully, within the child's ability to understand.

- Give simple explanations; there is no need to be complicated or elaborate.

- Use correct language (e.g., "He died," not "He passed away").

- Avoid euphemisms that may result in detrimental fears (e.g., "She is asleep," "God took her," "Mother has gone on a long trip").

- Assure the child that he or she is loved and will be taken care of, even though a sad thing has happened.

- Encourage the child to talk about thoughts and feelings.

- Permit the child to decide whether or not to go to the funeral.

- Expect the child to talk or participate only when he or she wishes to do so.

- Expect that a child's expression of grief will be intermittent.

- Share pictures and talk about the good times that have been enjoyed with the dying person.

# HOSPICE ROLE IN FACILITATING GRIEF PROCESS

## Goals of Grief Counseling

As discussed previously, grief in reaction to loss is normal. Past generations were consistently exposed to death in the home and usually had the benefit of close family and community support. However, supportive families and strong church and social ties are not as commonplace as they were, and many people do have difficulty coping with losses. Grieving must be experienced personally—it is not something that one person can do for another.

Worden (1991) proposes ten principles of counseling to facilitate uncomplicated or normal grief:

1. Help the survivor actualize the loss

2. Help the survivor to identify and express feelings

## Table 6.6 Children's Developmental Stages and Concepts of Death

**AGES 0–2**

There is no real concept of death. Egotistical thinking and dependency make these children vulnerable to fear of abandonment. Their need is for usual and ordinary needs to be met and to have someone present.

**AGES 3–4**

Death may be thought of as temporary (e.g., flowers die in the winter but come back in the spring). Children at this age may see death as mutilation if they have seen a dead animal by the road.

**AGES 5–7**

Death can be comprehended as a permanent event versus a temporary absence.

**AGES 8–11**

The idea of death's permanence becomes solidified, more like the adult concept, but fears of mutilation and abandonment may be present. Children at this age can associate religious ideas of heaven and hell.

**ADOLESCENCE**

In this complex stage of coping with personal life stresses, identity, and so forth, youth will be torn between coping with a death and getting back to their current problems. They may be tempted to regress to childhood behaviors. Sometimes they withdraw, and sometimes they overreact.

3. Assist living without the deceased

4. Facilitate emotional withdrawal from the deceased

5. Provide time to grieve

6. Interpret "normal" grief behavior

7. Allow for individual differences

8. Provide continuing support

9. Examine defenses and coping styles

10. Identify pathology and refer

Worden's principles are excellent guidelines for hospice grief counseling, perhaps the most important being to recognize when referral to a professional therapist is indicated.

## Therapeutic Approaches

The hospice role can be played out in different ways. The counseling role may be one of education, advocacy, or merely attentive presence. Provision of information is sometimes all it takes to help survivors begin the process of self-management or become empowered to seek available resources. Being an advocate with other professionals, family members, or community agencies may facilitate survivors' recovery during a period when they are incapable of speaking up for themselves. Attentive presence, specifically active listening, is a way caregivers can facilitate activation of grievers' own coping.

Following are some practical points to keep in mind:

◆ Permit tears—they are a natural reaction to grief and a healthy release of emotions.

◆ Permit and encourage expressions of pain and agony; phrases like "be brave" are not therapeutic—they imply a suffer-in-silence value.

◆ Encourage individuals to list things they did for the deceased when they berate themselves for "not having done enough."

◆ Patiently listen as the detailed story of the death is repeated over and over; this is part of actualizing the loss.

◆ Remember you are not the answer to the person's grief; you facilitate the person's own coping as he or she verbalizes thoughts.

◆ Be comfortable with not having an answer for every question asked, such as "Why me?" or "Why is God punishing me?"

◆ Encourage the griever to pay attention to personal needs; suggest that it is OK to take a respite from grief.

◆ Maintain an appropriate psychological distance—close enough to share the suffering but not so close as to be tempted to succumb to the despair.

◆ Listen with an open mind; never respond with judgment or interpretation.

◆ Encourage the griever to talk realistically about the deceased and their relationship.

◆ Assist the griever to identify problems or unfinished business that needs to be addressed.

## A Typical Hospice Bereavement Follow-Up Plan

Both the National Hospice Organization and Medicare hospice requirements mandate a program of bereavement care following the death of a patient. The commitment to the care of the patient's family and loved ones is a unique aspect of hospice care. A bereavement program can include individual and family counseling support groups, educational materials that describe normal grief and mourning, spiritual counseling, cards and notes, and telephone support. Knowing that a caring team will continue to follow their loved ones comforts many patients.

Bereavement services may be performed by anyone on the hospice team, but most hospices have a designated bereavement coordinator who provides these services, often with the help of volunteers. The length of time a particular person is followed is usually a year, and contact generally involves the following:

- Some contact the first few days and/or presence at the funeral or memorial service

- Availability by phone for a panic attack

- Periodic contacts, perhaps at 1 month, 3 months, 6 months, and 1 year

- Remembrance (card, phone call, or visit) on holidays or anniversaries

- A system for scheduling the follow-up contacts

- Documentation of contacts, ideally with an evaluation of grief resolution

- Method of feedback to the hospice team and subsequent referrals when indicated

- In some cases, planning and attendance at an annual memorial service

There is no timetable for the grief process. Rather, it can be characterized as a process of two steps forward and one step back. Hospice professionals assess the functioning of the bereaved with the goal of determining whether progress, albeit slow progress, is being made.

## REFERENCES AMD SUGGESTED READINGS

Byock, I. R. (1996). The nature of suffering and the nature of opportunity at the end of life. *Clinical Geriatric Medicine, 12*(2), 237–252.

Corless, I. B., Germino, B. B., & Pittman, M. A. (1995a). *A challenge for living: Dying, death and bereavement.* Boston: Jones and Bartlett.

Corless, I. B., Germino, B. B., & Pittman, M. A. (1995b). *Dying, death, and bereavement: Theoretical perspectives and other ways of knowing.* Boston: Jones and Bartlett.

Davidson, G. W. (1984). *Understanding mourning.* Minneapolis: Augsburg.

Freud, E. L. (1961). (Ed.). *Letters of Sigmund Freud.* New York: Basic Books.

Graham, J. (1982). *In the company of others: Understanding the human needs of cancer patients.* New York: Harcourt Brace Jovanovich.

Grollman, E. A. (1977). *Living when a loved one has died.* Boston: Beacon Press.

Holmes, T. H., & Rahe, R.H. (1967). The Social Readjustment Rating Scale. *Journal of Psychosomatic Research, 11,* 213–218.

Huber, R., & Gibson, J. W. (1990). New evidence for anticipatory grief. *The Hospice Journal, 6*(1), 49–67.

Kübler-Ross, E. (1975). *Death: The final stage of growth.* Englewood Cliffs, NJ: Prentice Hall.

Maslow, A. (1954). *Motivation and personality.* New York: Hemisphere.

Parkes, C. M. (1970). The first year of bereavement: A longitudinal study of the reaction of London widows to death of husbands. *Psychiatry, 33,*444–467.

Parkes, C. M., & Weiss, R. S. (1983). *Recovery from bereavement.* New York: Basic Books.

Rando, T. A. (1984). *Grief, dying, and death: Clinical interventions for caregivers.* Champaign, IL: Research Press.

Rando, T. A. (1993). *Treatment of complicated mourning.* Champaign, IL: Research Press.

Rando, T. A. (2000). The six dimensions of anticipatory mourning. In T. A. Rando (Ed.), *Clinical dimensions of anticipatory mourning: Theory and practice in working with the dying, their loved ones, and their caregivers.* Champaign, IL: Research Press.

Shuchter, S. R., & Zisook, S. (1986). Treatment of spousal bereavement: A multidimensional approach. *Psychiatric Annals, 16,* 295–305.

Volkan, V. D. (1985). Complicated mourning. *Annual of Psychoanalysis, 12,* 323–348.

Worden, J. W. (1991). *Grief counseling and grief therapy* (2nd ed.). New York: Springer.

# CHAPTER 7

# Spiritual Care

**PURPOSE**

The purpose of this chapter is to describe spiritual pain, discuss its assessment, and present guidelines for therapeutic interventions.

**OBJECTIVES**

Upon completion of this chapter, the learner will be able to:

1. Define spiritual pain

2. Explain the difference between religious and spiritual needs

3. List some therapeutic interventions in this area

**CONTENT OUTLINE**

I. Overview of Spiritual Needs

    A. Introduction

    B. Difference between religious and spiritual needs

    C. Universal spiritual needs

II. Assessment of Spiritual Needs

    A. Approaching the patient

    B. Assessment tools

III. Planning Spiritual Care Interventions

    A. Therapeutic techniques

    B. Openness and flexibility in response to patient and family

# OVERVIEW OF SPIRITUAL NEEDS

## Introduction

Inclusion of spiritual care in the care of dying persons has a long tradition, from medieval days to Dr. Cicely Saunders' focus on its importance in the earliest days of hospice. In medieval times, ministry to the sick and needy was performed by religious figures who felt it their duty. When Dr. Saunders established St. Christopher's Hospice in England, she emphasized the need to address emotional and spiritual distresses as well as physical distresses (Du Boulay, 1984). Today, spiritual care is an essential part of the hospice effort as well as a requirement of the Joint Commission on Accreditation of Health Care Organizations, the National Hospice Organization, and Medicare. Comprehensive care in terminal illness must include an assessment and plan of care for spiritual distresses or dysfunction.

Just as some patients may not experience or report serious overt physical pain, some patients may not express any overt spiritual pain. However, many patients will experience pain in their inner being that can be a greater deterrent to comfort than any physical pain. Spiritual pain is definitely a factor in total suffering. Rather than being expressed by outward acts, *spirituality* involves the moral consciousness or soul and includes thinking, motivation, and feeling. If an individual is dissatisfied in his or her inner being, there will be spiritual distresses. Inner anguish is frequently expressed as physical symptoms because this may be easier than "baring one's soul."

## Difference between Religious and Spiritual Needs

It is important to recognize the distinction between spiritual needs and religious needs, with spirituality being a broader concept, reflecting more universal expectations. Religious needs generally relate to the dogma, practices, and rituals of worship of specific organized groups. They include the following:

- Prayers, meditation
- Scripture or other readings
- Sacraments, communion
- Confession, penance
- Worship services
- Clergy visits, pastoral counseling
- Anointing

Whereas religion deals with practices and rituals, the spiritual part of human life refers to the inner self and its relationship to the universe and a higher power. It is the part of human experience dealing with the meaning of life, with death, and with what happens after we die. It is hard to define spirituality because it is intangible and transcends measurable sensory phenomenon. Usually, spiritual contentment is equated with having found meaning in life, experiencing self-worth, and feeling at peace with relationships. When death seems imminent, it is common for suppressed or ignored spiritual concerns to emerge. Every individual will express these needs in a different way. Some people find solace in rituals alone, others will express the need to explore spiritual concerns, many will want to engage in both, and some will ignore the subject altogether.

## Universal Spiritual Needs

Religious beliefs and denominational affiliations differ widely; however, it is important to recognize universal spiritual needs. Individuals vary in how they see the world and their relationship to it, as well as in their ideas about creation, deity, meaning of life, and what happens at death. There are, however, certain basic human spiritual needs frequently seen in dying patients, regardless of culture or religion. These universal spiritual needs are listed in Table 7.1.

# ASSESSMENT OF SPIRITUAL NEEDS

## Approaching the Patient

Terminal illness precipitates numerous problems to be resolved, and time may be short, so it is essential for all team members to use the skills of observation, communication, and sensitivity to facilitate expression of spiritual needs. The evaluation should be ongoing, especially because the patient may be reluctant to share emotional issues until trust is established. The following considerations may be useful during spiritual and religious assessment:

- ◆ Not all patients or significant others will be able to share their troubling thoughts.

- ◆ Spiritual assessment can be thought of as evaluation of relational well-being.

- ◆ Given that spiritual assessment and spiritual care must be ongoing and available when the patient is ready, the entire interdisciplinary team must participate.

## Table 7.1 Universal Spiritual Needs

**NEED FOR BELONGING AND RELATIONSHIPS**

> To be cared for, not abandoned or isolated
>
> To give and receive love
>
> For comfort and peace
>
> Relationship needs: family, significant others, deity

**NEED TO EXPLORE MEANING OF LIFE, SUFFERING, AND DEATH**

> To experience affirmation of self-worth
>
> For acceptance: of self, of others, of human events
>
> To recognize sources of strength to face death
>
> To contemplate what gives a sense of purpose and fulfillment
>
> To discover personal meaning of pain and death
>
> To redefine hopes and goals
>
> To move on to detachment and solitude

**NEED FOR RECONCILIATION**

> To acknowledge unfinished/unresolved conflicts
>
> To recognize nagging resentment and bitterness
>
> To recognize feelings of guilt and blame
>
> To be able to forgive and accept forgiveness

- The patient's right to privacy must be honored in this area of care, just as in any physical or psychosocial context.
- Assessment should discover the patient's inner resources for dealing with dying.
- Staff should be alert to spiritual pain, even if it is not verbalized.
- Diverse belief systems and even more diverse individual interpretations will exist, even within a family unit, sometimes resulting in intense conflicts.
- Evaluation may change as illness progresses; when faced with impending death, some patients will find themselves returning to earlier beliefs and values.

## Assessment Tools

There should be a specific plan for this type of assessment. Reaching a consensus among hospice team members on the best approach to assessment and intervention may be a challenge, but it is necessary.

Engaging in life review is a nonthreatening way to begin assessing belief systems and unresolved issues. A patient's stories about the future can be helpful for assessing hope and fear. Spiritual assessments and psychosocial assessments complement each other and can easily be combined.

In one hospice program, after using various assessment approaches, team members decided on a set of questions that they thought would be nonthreatening, would get to the heart of spiritual issues, and would not be embarrassing for the staff or the patient. The questions were then used as their spiritual assessment tool:

- How would you describe your philosophy of life?

- What nourishes your spirit?

- What is your source of strength when you feel afraid or need special help?

- What is your belief about death and/or an afterlife?

- What is especially meaningful or frightening to you now?

- Are there unresolved issues such as resentment, guilt, anger, anxiety, or bitterness that you wish to discuss with someone?

- Do you want us to contact a particular clergy person whom you would want to pay you a visit?

# PLANNING SPIRITUAL CARE INTERVENTIONS

## Therapeutic Techniques

- Offer presence as a comfort and an opportunity for communication. Anything said or done during this time must be compatible with the beliefs and values of the patient. Encourage family or significant others to sit with the patient, even if nothing is said.

- Arrange clergy visitation as desired by the patient.

- Listen to stories or life reviews. Doing so is an excellent way to bring out contributions and accomplishments, validate the person's value to self or others, and explore spiritual issues.

- Allow expressions of anger, guilt, hurt, and fear without minimizing or explaining away; the patient may need encouragement to acknowledge the feelings and then let them go.

- Avoid clichés such as "It is God's will," "Time heals all wounds," "God wants him in heaven," and so forth. Such messages may not match the patient's beliefs. Never say, "Everything's going to be all right" or "You shouldn't feel that way."

♦ Read scriptures or other materials as desired by the patient.

♦ Encourage appropriate joy and humor. Laughter brings a lift to the spirit, as well as serving to celebrate life and keep things in perspective.

♦ Share prayers, meditation, or music if the patient desires them.

♦ Use massage and relaxation to help the patient relax and be better able to deal with disturbing spiritual matters. These techniques may also help to control pain and other distressing symptoms.

♦ Assist the patient in reframing goals so that they are attainable and meaningful. Sometimes this means exploring strengths, priorities, and past experiences.

## Openness and Flexibility in Response to Patient and Family

All hospice programs should recognize and be open to spiritual and religious diversity. This goal is best stated in the United Nations' (1981) *Declaration on the Elimination of All Forms of Intolerance and of Discrimination Based on Religion and Belief:*

> Everyone shall have the right to freedom of thought, conscience and religion. This right shall include freedom to have a religion or whatever belief of his choice, and freedom, either individually or in community with others and in public or private, to manifest his religion or belief in worship, observance, practice and teaching. (p. 3)

Because palliative care is concerned with the well-being of the whole person, spiritual and religious aspects must be an integral part of care. There must be full respect for patients' concepts of deity, values, and beliefs, as well as acceptance of their right to discuss or not discuss these issues with staff. Team members should never impose their personal beliefs. Those patients who wish to participate in spiritual or religious activities should be enabled to do so. Supportive interventions must be offered in ways that are nonsectarian, nondogmatic, and in keeping with patients' own views of the world.

Many patients, consciously or subconsciously, will find the dying process an opportunity for personal growth. Spiritual solutions cannot always be offered. Caregivers should view all interactions about the spiritual realm as opportunities to facilitate coping skills, as is the case for psychosocial problems. When hospice staff show a caring attitude and are open to spiritual aspects, the potential for patients' inner healing is greatly enhanced.

## REFERENCES AND SUGGESTED READINGS

Amenta, M. O. (1986). Spiritual concerns. In M. O. Amenta & N. L. Bohnet (Eds.), *Nursing care of the terminally ill.* Boston: Little, Brown.

Dossey, L. (1989). *Recovering the soul: A scientific and spiritual search.* New York: Bantam Books.

Du Boulay, S. (1984). *Cicely Saunders: The founder of the modern hospice movement.* London, England: Hodder and Stoughton.

Dudley, J. R., Smith, C., & Millison, M. B. (1995). Unfinished business: Assessing the spiritual needs of hospice clients. *American Journal of Hospice and Palliative Care, 12*(2), 30–37.

Fish, S., & Shelly, J. (Eds.). (1983). *Spiritual care* (2nd ed.). Downers Grove, IL: Inter-Varsity Press.

Gates, G. N. (1987). Where is the pastoral counselor in the hospice movement? *Journal of Pastoral Care, 41,* 32–38.

Hay, M. W. (1989). Principles in building spiritual assessment tools. *American Journal of Hospice Care, 6*(5), 25–31.

Irion, P. C. (1984). *Hospice and ministry.* Nashville: Parthenon Press.

Kaczorowski, J. M. (1989). Spiritual well being and anxiety in adults diagnosed with cancer. *The Hospice Journal, 5*(3–4), 105–116.

Karnes, B. (1987). Spiritual moment of death. *American Journal of Hospice Care, 4*(5), 28–29.

Kaye, P. (1990). *Symptom control in hospice and palliative care.* Essex, CT: Hospice Education Institute.

Millison, M. B. (1988). Spirituality and the caregiver: Developing an underutilized facet of care. *American Journal of Hospice Care, 5*(2), 37–44.

Millison, M. B., & Dudley, J. R. (1992). Providing spiritual support: A job for all hospice professionals. *The Hospice Journal, 8*(4), 49–66.

O'Brien, P. (1992). Social work and spirituality: Clarifying the concept for practice. *Spirituality and Social Work Journal, 3*(1), 2–5.

O'Connor, P. (1988). The role of spiritual care in hospice. *American Journal of Hospice Care, 5*(4), 31–37.

Pumphrey, J. B. (1982). Spiritual and religious aspects. In B. Cassileth & P. Cassileth (Eds.), *Clinical care of the terminal cancer patient.* Philadelphia: Lea & Febiger.

Satterly, L. R. (1993). *Tattooed in the cradle.* Maple Glen, PA: The SEARCH Foundation.

Speck, P. W. (1993). Spiritual issues in palliative care. In D. Doyle, G. W. C. Hanks, & N. MacDonald (Eds.), *Oxford textbook of palliative medicine.* New York: Oxford University Press.

Spiritual Care Work Group of the International Work Group on Death, Dying, and Bereavement. (1990). Assumptions and principles of spiritual care. *Death Studies, 14*(1), 75–81.

United Nations. (1981). *Declaration on the elimination of all forms of intolerance and of discrimination based on religion and belief.* New York: Author.

Wald, F. S. (1989). The widening scope of spiritual care. *American Journal of Hospice Care, 6*(4) 40–43.

# CHAPTER 8

# Pain Management

**PURPOSE**

The purpose of this chapter is to outline the principles of appropriate relief of pain symptoms exhibited by patients who have a terminal illness. Good pain management is essential to optimize quality of life and ease physical, social, and spiritual pain.

**OBJECTIVES**

Upon completion of this chapter, the learner will be able to:

1. Identify pain as a complex entity with multiple treatment modalities

2. Define barriers and myths concerning pain management

3. State the major principles of pain assessment and pain management

**CONTENT OUTLINE**

I. Scope of the Pain Problem

   A.  Incidence and definitions

   B.  Multifactorial etiologies

   C.  Separating myth from reality

   D.  Barriers to pain management

   E.  Types of pain

   F.  Origins of pain

II. Assessing and Treating Pain

   A.  Pain assessment techniques

B. Treatment strategies

1. The WHO approach

2. Choosing drugs

3. Changing drugs or route of administration

4. Calculating the breakthrough dose

5. Adjuvant medications

6. Nonpharmacologic measures

7. Drugs to avoid

# SCOPE OF THE PAIN PROBLEM

## Incidence and Definitions

According to Spross (1990) and others, widespread undertreatment of pain in terminal illness continues despite great knowledge about the topic. According to the report of the Institute of Medicine's (1997) Committee on Care at the End of Life, if physician and hospital performance in infection control were as poor as pain management is, there would be a national outcry for change. It is estimated that 70 to 90% of patients with advanced disease experience pain and that close to 100% of that pain can be controlled with readily available medications and techniques. It has become the mission of those working in hospice care to achieve relief of pain and provide comfort in the last days, freeing the patient to deal with other matters of personal concern.

*Pain* may be defined as an unpleasant sensory and emotional experience associated with actual or potential tissue damage. A more clinically applicable definition is that of McCaffery and Beebe (1989), who say that pain is what the patient says it is. It should always be regarded as totally subjective (i.e., defined by the person experiencing it). Table 8.1 gives definitions for a number of terms helpful in discussing pain.

The caregiver's challenge is to assess persistently all potential contributing factors. The nature of pain is complex. It is important to understand the biopsychosocial and spiritual dimensions of suffering and be prepared to address each of them to be effective in pain management.

## Multifactorial Etiologies

As noted, and as shown in the figure on page 106, pain is a complex phenomenon. Biological issues include the nature of the pain and the

## Table 8.1   Terms Relevant in the Discussion of Pain

***Addiction:*** A psychological and social syndrome characterized by compulsion to seek and take drugs for other than their therapeutic effect.

***Pseudoaddiction:*** A common iatrogenic syndrome in which patients develop certain behavioral characteristics of psychological dependence as a result of inadequate pain treatment.

***Tolerance:*** The pharmacologic phenomenon in which increasing doses of the same drug are required to achieve the same therapeutic effect.

***Dependence:*** Physiological adaptation of the body to the presence of an opioid. This means side effects are tolerated but also that doses must be titrated downward slowly if drug is to be discontinued in order to prevent withdrawal symptoms (nausea, vomiting, cramps, diaphoresis, chills).

***Allodynia:*** Pain from a stimulus that does not normally evoke pain, such as contact with bed linens or touching the skin with a piece of cotton or an ice cube.

***Dysesthesia:*** Impairment of sense of touch, accompanied by pain similar to allodynia.

***Hyperpathia:*** An abnormally painful reaction, usually with explosive onset and great severity.

***Hypoalgesia/hyperalgesia:*** Diminished/increased pain in response to a normally painful stimulus.

***Paresthesia:*** Abnormal sensations such as tingling, burning, or tightness.

***Suffering:*** A complex physical, psychological, social, and spiritual process.

type of disease invading the body. For example, patients with extensive cancer have pain resulting from extension into soft tissues, visceral or bone involvement, nerve compression or destruction, and increased intracranial pressure. There may also be pain resulting from cancer treatments, such as chronic postoperative scar pain, stomatitis from chemotherapy, or cystitis from radiation therapy. Pain can be secondary to aspects of decreased functional status such as bedsores, constipation, or muscle spasms. Psychologically, the patient may be distressed by loss of autonomy, dependence on others, concern over finances, and, particularly, loss of self-esteem and self-actualization. Social issues include concerns about the caregiver's health, about

## Multifactorial Influences on Pain Perception

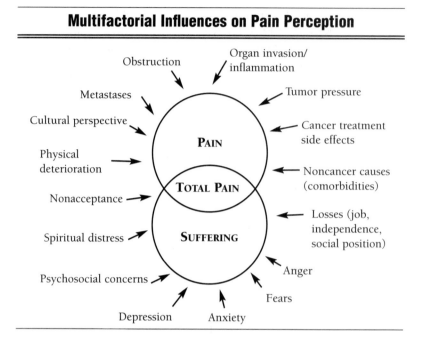

being a burden, and about individual family dynamics. Spiritual pain, inner conflicts related to values and religious beliefs, may be equally distressing. Cultural background will influence how one interprets and reacts to pain.

The management of the pain of terminal disease cannot be achieved with pharmacologic means alone. Because pain is a totally subjective experience and because patients with limited life expectancy have many factors that contribute to their interpretation of pain—social and financial concerns, fear of dying, guilt, perceived need to suffer—the use of drugs should be in addition to, and not instead of, a thorough holistic assessment and interdisciplinary interventions.

## Separating Myth from Reality

Relief of pain in the terminal patient permits the patient to be more active, possibly more ambulatory, and more involved in self-care and activities of daily living. It also frees the patient to address family, spiritual, or other psychosocial concerns, impossible when one is consumed with pain.

Most often, in traditional medical and surgical settings, we focus on acute pain, treating it conservatively to avoid possible addiction to opioids. Many practitioners, therefore, are unaware of the large body of research begun by Dr. Cicely Saunders in London and continued on by Twycross (1994), Houde (1979), Melzack (1990), Fields

(1987), Portenoy (Portenoy, 1989; Portenoy & Hagen, 1990; Portenoy & Kanner, 1996), Foley (1993), and others. These studies have shown that many terminally ill patients may need, and can tolerate, very large doses of opioids for pain relief. They do not become addicted, their lives are not shortened, and opioids rarely, if ever, cause respiratory depression. For clinicians, patients, and families, it is necessary to dispel some of the old myths and misconceptions.

**Myth:** Narcotics cause addiction.

**Reality:** A person with physiologic pain doesn't experience addiction but rather tolerance (resistance to side effects) and physical dependence (requiring an increased dose secondary to physiological adaptation).

**Myth:** Narcotics depress respirations.

**Reality:** Most patients in pain have increased rates of respiration; relief of pain permits a decrease to a more normal rate. In a study by Grond, Zech, Schugs, Lynch, and Lehman (1991), no patient developed subnormal respirations regardless of opioid dose. Pain antagonizes the respiratory depressant effects of opiates so that, when medication is carefully titrated, opiate depression of respiration is uncommon.

**Myth:** Morphine should be saved for the end.

**Reality:** Morphine is an effective analgesic that should be used when less potent drugs do not work. Some patients do well on very low doses.

**Myth:** Start cautiously because there is a limit to dose.

**Reality:** There is no ceiling or maximum recommended dose for full opioid agonists, and, in fact, very large doses of morphine (e.g., several hundred milligrams every 4 hours), may be needed for severe pain.

**Myth:** If heroin were legalized, it would solve our problems.

**Reality:** We already have every advantage of heroin in morphine because morphine is what heroin breaks down into; we just need to use properly what we already have.

**Myth:** Having narcotics around the house will tempt addicts to steal from me.

**Reality:** There is always some potential for criminal activity, but most patients use oral and/or sustained-release medications; generally, addicts do not use drugs in these forms. The incidence of diversion of drugs prescribed for terminal patients is very low.

## Barriers to Pain Management

The two most common barriers to good pain management are inadequate knowledge and fear of addiction or side effects. Lack of knowledge extends to the use of appropriate assessments and effective opioid dosing. Some fear of reprisal from state and federal regulators may also exist concerning the volume of narcotics prescribed by individual physicians. This is especially true in states with "triplicate" laws—meaning prescriptions are written in triplicate for purposes of tracking individual doctors' patterns of prescribing.

Sometimes patients or family members are reluctant to report pain or reluctant to take or give prescribed medications. The reasons may vary from personal fears of addiction to religious or financial concerns. Patients may want to appear as "good" and noncomplaining, and are thus reluctant to express their pain. Patients and families may think that taking morphine means the end is near and so must be resisted. Finally, lack of insurance coverage or financial resources may prohibit medical attention or purchase of medications.

## Types of Pain

It is important to recognize different types of pain because the treatment will differ for each. The following definitions are useful: *Acute pain* results from injury to the body, dissipating as healing occurs. It serves a purpose and is limited in time. It is often accompanied by autonomic nervous system activity such as tachycardia, hypertension, diaphoresis, pallor, and so on. Pain from a burn, appendicitis, surgery, or a broken bone is of this sort. *Chronic pain* is persistent pain serving no useful purpose. Because it is rarely accompanied by autonomic nervous system activity, inexperienced clinicians may doubt the validity of the pain complaint. The most common example we see in hospice is in end-stage cancer. Chronic pain may originate from somatic, visceral, or neuritic sources.

Acute or episodic pain would be treated with as-needed (PRN) dosing. Any pain that is chronic (i.e., present most of the time) would be treated with around-the-clock dosing. Chronic pain with around-the-clock dosing should always have a PRN dose order for breakthrough pain. There also will be patients who have chronic pain but who occasionally will have acute pain unrelated to the terminal diagnosis, such as a migraine headache. Another example is a bed-bound patient whose around-the-clock medication for the persistent pain of bone metastasis is adequate except for certain movements, such as a bed bath or turning in bed. This patient would need a PRN dose prior to such painful activity.

## Origins of Pain

Pain has many origins. *Nociceptive pain* is related to noxious sensations resulting from mechanical, thermal, or chemical stimulation of intact afferent nerve fibers. The noxious stimuli cause tissue damage, resulting in the release of nociceptive substances such as serotonin, substance P, bradykinins, histamines, and prostaglandins. The two types of nociceptive pain are somatic and visceral. *Somatic pain* results from direct stimulation to intact afferent nerve endings in skin, bone, and connective tissues. It is characterized by dull or sharp, gnawing, aching, and well-localized pain. *Visceral pain* results from direct stimulation to intact afferent nerve endings in viscera, or organs with hollow cavities such as the stomach, bowel, esophagus, or small intestines. It is described as pressure, cramping, and fullness, and is of nonspecific location. These types of pain generally respond well to opioid analgesics. Because nonsteroidal anti-inflammatory drugs (NSAIDs) block the formation of these pain-stimulating substances peripherally, they are a great asset to pain management in addition to opioids.

Neuropathic pain is caused by peripheral or central nervous system (CNS) nerve injury, characterized by burning, stabbing, shooting, and tingling pain, and associated with allodynia, paresthesias, and dysesthesias. Examples of conditions generating such pain are postradiation radiculitis, acute herpes zoster, postherpetic neuralgia, phantom-limb pain, nerve injury due to surgical incision, and tumor pressure or invasion of nerve plexuses. Neuropathic pain does not respond well to opioid analgesics, but it usually does respond well to tricyclic antidepressants and anticonvulsants.

# ASSESSING AND TREATING PAIN

## Pain Assessment Techniques

Proper assessment must precede administration of analgesics. Ascertaining the following information *after* knowing the patient's medical conditions will lead to effective interventions without undertreatment, overtreatment, or inappropriate treatment. It is essential to know the patient's personal values as well: One patient may prefer to have a little pain if it means being a little more alert. Another patient may prefer sleeping all the time rather than having any pain at all. Assessment should always include the following, initially and on an ongoing basis.

### Description of pain

Ask: "What does it feel like?" Look for descriptor words, clues to the origin of pain.

- Somatic pain: Dull, gnawing, aching, sharp, well-located
- Visceral pain: Pressure, feeling of fullness, nonspecific location
- Neuropathic pain: Lancinating, burning, shooting, like an electrical shock

### Location of pain

Ask: "Where is the pain, and does it go anywhere else?" Common patterns of referred pain are as follows:

- Stomach, esophagus, pancreas, and retroperitoneal disease (to the back)
- Gallbladder (to the scapula)
- Retrosigmoid (to the sacrum/rectum)
- Liver (to the right shoulder)

### Severity or intensity of pain

Ask: "How bad is the pain?"

- The most common scale is 1 to 10, with 10 being the worst possible pain. Use this scale to assess current pain, when pain is greatest/least, and 1 hour after analgesia.
- Determine the patient's perception of acceptable pain level.
- Establish what factors affect the pain ("What makes it better? Worse?").
- Effectiveness of current and past treatments
- What medications have been tried?
- Which medications worked best?
- Which nonmedicinal treatments help?

### Limitations caused by pain

- Activity?
- Sleep?
- Mood?
- Significance of limitations to the patient?

### Ongoing reassessment

- With new or increased pain, review all of the preceding.

- Facilitate ongoing assessment by using flow sheets or patient diaries.

- Consistently use the same scale for measuring pain intensity in each patient.

## Treatment Strategies

### The WHO Approach

The World Health Organization (WHO, 1990) has suggested effective approaches to management of cancer pain. These approaches are appropriate for all chronic pain in terminal care.

### *By mouth*

- Use the simplest modality; if the patient can swallow, the oral route is most appropriate.

- A combination of sustained release (SR) and immediate release (IR) medications works well orally.

- When the patient cannot swallow, rectal, sublingual, buccal, or transdermal routes may be used.

### *By the clock*

- Constant pain requires constant dosing.

- Around-the-clock dosing with PRN doses for any breakthrough pain maintains a constant level of drug and quality pain control.

### *By the ladder*

- The goal is to provide the right drug, at the right dose, at the right frequency.

- Patients do not necessarily start on Step 1. Patients who have moderate-to-severe pain when first seen should be started at Step 2 or Step 3 of the ladder.

- The WHO ladder matches degree of pain to strength of drugs. Think of Step 1 as acetaminophen or equivalents for mild pain, Step 2 as codeine or equivalents for moderate pain, and Step 3 as morphine or equivalents for severe pain. At any level, analgesic adjuvants may be useful.

### *For the individual*

- What helps one person may not help another.

- The patient may have previous experience, aversions, allergies.

- Individuals vary in degree of side effects; nausea and vomiting are easily treated, respiratory depression is rare, sedation or mental clouding may require evaluation and treatment, and a bowel regime to prevent constipation should be routine on every patient on opioids.
- Pain is subjective: It is what the patient says it is.

### With attention to detail

- Intervals on PRN orders should match duration of action.
- Always add a bowel regime.
- Constantly reassess to note changes, new symptoms, and comorbidities other than the life-threatening illness.
- Non-opioid analgesics can be very effective for mild to moderate pain and can enhance pain management when given with opioids because they act peripherally (blocking the formation of bradykinins, prostaglandins, etc.), whereas opioids act centrally. This combination is effective in bone pain.
- Because pain is a natural antagonist to the analgesic, respiratory depression is rarely seen.
- Pain should be thought of as the fifth vital sign for all patients with chronic pain. Some facilities make this a part of the vital signs flow sheet.
- Placebos should never be used to test the pain problem.
- Opioid tolerance and physical dependence do not equate to addiction.
- If the pain is not satisfactorily relieved, some change should be made to dosage, choice of drug, adjuvants, psychosocial/spiritual therapies, or other areas.
- If the pain is satisfactorily relieved by the current dosing but consistently recurs before the next dose, the interval needs to be shortened.
- Sustained release pills should never be crushed.
- When using the fentanyl transdermal (Duragesic) patch, remember that it takes 12 to 18 hours to reach peak dose absorption, so the previous drug should be continued for the first 12 hours or PRN doses should be ordered.

### Choosing Drugs

Table 8.2 illustrates some of the many analgesic options available for different levels of pain. It is important to remember that a different drug in the same category may be effective before going to a stronger category. One must be cautious with NSAIDs, combination products, and codeine products because there are ceiling doses. *Ceiling dose* means the maximum dose giving therapeutic results without undesirable side effects. For example, acetaminophen (Tylenol) has a ceiling dose of 4 g (4,000 mg) because of potential liver damage. Although they may not have ceiling doses, other analgesics may be limited due to side effects. NSAIDs are limited because of associated gastrointestinal distress. Aspirin is limited because of potential bleeding problems. Codeine products may need to be limited because of constipation, sedation, hallucinations, and other effects.

Whether considering the around-the-clock dose or the PRN breakthrough dose, the dosing schedule should agree with the duration of action of the drug being used. Table 8.3 demonstrates some durations of action for drugs commonly used in terminal care.

> *A word of caution: The information in the following pages is given only to provide a general context for understanding the pharmaceutical treatment of pain. All treatments must be chosen on an individual basis and medications prescribed per the pharmaceutical company's current dosing recommendations.*

## Changing Drugs or Route of Administration

If the status of the patient changes and it becomes prudent to switch from oral to some other method of administration, or vice versa, we must know the relative analgesic potencies. This is sometimes referred to as *equianalgesic dosing*, meaning that all analgesics do not have the same potency, milligram for milligram, nor do they absorb equally well via oral to parenteral routes. Table 8.4 shows relative, or equal, potencies of different drugs, and potencies of the same drug by different routes, to maintain the same level of analgesic effectiveness. All doses on the chart are equivalent to 10 milligrams of morphine sulfate administered parenterally.

Following is the method suggested by the American Pain Society (APS, 1999) for calculating changes:

1. Total the current 24-hour dose of the drug used (calculate separately if more than one drug used).

2. Divide that number by the equianalgesic number on the table for the current drug and route of administration. This gives you the number of morphine equivalents the patient is taking.

# Table 8.2   Analgesics

## NON-OPIOIDS

| BRAND | GENERIC NAME | USUAL DOSAGE | COMMENTS |
|---|---|---|---|
| (generic) | Aspirin | 325–650 mg q4h | Not to exceed 4 g/d |
| Tylenol | Acetaminophen | 325–650 mg q4h | Not to exceed 4 g/d |
| Trilisate | Choline-magnesium salicylate | 1,000 mg BID or TID | |
| Voltaren | Diclofenac | 50 mg TID | |
| Dolobid | Diflunisal | 250 mg BID or TID | |
| Lodine | Etodolac | 200–400 mg q6–8h | Not to exceed 1,200 mg/d |
| Motrin, Advil, Nuprin | Ibuprofen | 200–400 mg q4–6h | Not to exceed 3.2 g/d |
| Indocin | Indomethacin | 50 mg BID or TID | Not to exceed 200 mg/d |
| Disalcid, Amigesic | Salsalate | 500 mg q4h | Not to exceed 3 g/d |

## MILD OPIOIDS

| BRAND | GENERIC NAME AND STRENGTHS (DOSE VARIES) | COMMENTS |
|---|---|---|
| Lorcet | Hydrocodone, 10 mg<br>Acetaminophen, 650 mg | |
| Lortab | Hydrocodone, 2.5, 5, or 7.5 mg<br>Acetaminophen, 500 mg | |
| Percocet | Oxycodone/acetaminophen, 2.5 mg/325 mg,<br>5 mg/325 mg, 7.5 mg/500 mg, 10 mg/650 mg | Tylox (brand) has 5 mg oxycodone and 500 mg acetaminophen |

114

| Brand | Generic Name and Strengths (dose varies) | Comments |
| --- | --- | --- |
| **Percodan** | Oxycodone HCl, 4.5 mg<br>Oxycodone terephthalate, 0.38 mg<br>Aspirin, 325 mg | |
| **Tylenol with codeine** | Codeine phosphate, 7.5, 15, 30, 60 mg<br>Acetaminophen, 300 mg | |
| **Vicodan** | Hydrocodone bitartrate, 5 mg, 7.5 mg<br>Acetaminophen, 500 mg, 750 mg | |
| **STRONG OPIOIDS** | | |
| **BRAND** | **GENERIC NAME AND STRENGTHS (DOSE VARIES)** | **COMMENTS** |
| **Dilaudid** | Hydromorphone HCl, 2, 4, or 8 mg | |
| **Levo-Dromoran** | Levorphanol tartrate, 2 mg | Caution: Long plasma half-life (12–16 h) |
| **MS Contin, Oramorph SR** | Morphine sulfate SR, 15, 30, 60, 100 mg | SR administered q12h |
| **Roxanol SR** | Morphine sulfate SR, 30 mg | SR administered q8h |
| **Kadian** | Morphine sulfate SR, 20, 50, 100 mg | SR administered q24h |
| **Roxanol MSIR** | Liquid morphine sulfate, varying strengths | Concentrates good for sublingual or buccal administration |
| **Roxanol RMS** | Morphine sulphate, in suppository form | |
| **Dolophine HCl** | Methadone, 5, 10 mg | Caution: Long half-life (24–36 h); also available in injectable and liquid forms |
| **Numorphan** | Oxymorphone, 1 or 1.5mg/ml, injectable | Also available in suppositories |
| **Duragesic** | Fentanyl citrate, transdermal patches, 25, 50, 75, 100 mcg/h | Administered q72h as skin patch; absorption varies with amount of fat tissue (may require q48h administration) |

BID = twice a day; HCl = hydrochloride; MS = morphine sulfate; MSIR = morphine sulfate immediate release; q_h = every _ hours; RMS = rectal morphine sulfate; SR = sustained release; TID = three times a day

## Table 8.3   Hours of Action for Commonly Used Drugs

Codeine . . . . . . . . . . . . . . . . . . . . . . . . . . . . . . . . . . . . . . . . . . . . . . . 4–6

Meperidine (Demerol) . . . . . . . . . . . . . . . . . . . . . . . . . . . . . . . . . 2–3

Hydromorphone (Dilaudid) . . . . . . . . . . . . . . . . . . . . . . . . . . . . 4–5

Methadone . . . . . . . . . . . . . . . . . . . . . . . . . . . . . . . . . . . . . . . . . . . . 6–8

Morphine immediate release . . . . . . . . . . . . . . . . . . . . . . . . . . . 2–4

Morphine sustained release . . . . . . . . . . . . . . . . . . . . . 8, 12, or 24

Fentanyl transdermal . . . . . . . . . . . . . . . . . . . . . . . . . . . . . . . . . . . 72
(or 48 if patient regularly has pain on third day)

3. Multiply the above number by the number for the new drug and route. This will give you the 24-hour dose for the new drug or route.

4. Divide the dose according to the frequency of administration. For example, if you plan to give the drug four times a day, you would divide the 24-hour total by 6.

**Calculating the Breakthrough Dose**

All patients who have persistent pain and are on around-the-clock dosing should have an additional order for a PRN dose for breakthrough or incidental pain. Also referred to as a "rescue" dose, it should be a short-acting drug. The APS recommends that the breakthrough dose be 10 to 15% of the 24-hour total dose, available every 2 hours if needed. Other leading pain experts vary in their recommendations, both in dose and frequency of administration, but the goal is to assure that adequate medication is ordered to keep the patient comfortable. Factors that may alter the percentage or frequency of dosing might be severity of the breakthrough pain (e.g., in the 2 to 4 range or the 7 to 9 range on the 10-point pain scale), the patient's past experience with breakthrough pain, frequency of occurrence, and the patient's degree of distress about the breakthrough pain. It is generally agreed that the baseline around-the-clock dose should be increased if the patient consistently uses three or more breakthrough doses in a 24-hour period.

**Adjuvant Medications**

Adjuvant drugs are those that may enhance the effects of the analgesics, have independent analgesic activity, counteract side effects of analgesics, or ameliorate symptoms that may contribute to the overall suffering. Adding an adjuvant may be more effective than simply continuing to increase an opioid. According to the Agency

## Table 8.4  Relative Analgesic Equivalents

| ANALGESIC | PARENTERAL DOSE | ORAL DOSE |
|---|---|---|
| Morphine | 10 mg | 30 mg |
| Codeine | 130 mg | 200 mg |
| Methadone | 10 mg | 20 mg |
| Hydromorphone (Dilaudid) | 1.5 mg | 7.5 mg |
| Levorphanol (Levo-Dromoran) | 2 mg | 4 mg |
| Meperidine (Demerol) | 100 mg | 300 mg |
| Oxycodone | — | 15 mg |
| Hydrocodone | — | 45 mg |
| Oxymorphone (Numorphan) | 1 mg | — |
| Fentanyl transdermal (Duragesic) | 0.1 mg | |

(Conversion: Half of the 24-hour morphine equivalent is the microgram-per-hour dose of fentanyl.)

for Health Care Policy and Research (1995) guidelines, adjuvant drugs are valuable during all phases of pain management to enhance analgesic efficacy, treat concurrent problems, and provide independent analgesia for specific types of pain. A general summary is offered in Table 8.5.

**Nonpharmacologic Measures**

Because pain is a totally subjective experience and is influenced by all manner of spiritual, cultural, social, psychological, and physical phenomena, it is reasonable to expect that more than one avenue exists to relieve distress. Aside from simply interacting with the patient in a positive manner, many physical and psychosocial approaches can be very effective. Although we must not be negligent in utilizing available and appropriate medications, we would be equally negligent if we continued to medicate without considering some extremely effective nonmedicinal measures. These include physical as well as psychosocial/spiritual modalities.

*Physical modalities*

- ◆ Position changes

- ◆ Heat or cold applications

- ◆ Massage

- ◆ Counterstimulation, such as transcutaneous electrical nerve stimulation (TENS) therapy or acupuncture

## Table 8.5  Adjuvant Medications

| Drug Type | Example | Indication |
|---|---|---|
| Tricyclic antidepressants | Amitriptyline, doxepin, imipramine, nortriptyline | Specific drug for neuropathic or phantom pain; relieves depression; helps insomnia. |
| Antianxiety drugs | Alprozolam, flurazepam, lorazepam, buspirone | Decreases stress, anxiety, insomnia. |
| Phenothiazines | Prochlorperazine, chlorpromazine | Effective antiemetic and anxiolytic. |
| Steroids | Prednisone, dexamethasone | Reduces tumor edema, especially useful with brain tumors. Also used for anorexia, but of limited value. |
| Antihistamines | Hydroxyzine | Mild anxiolytic; relieves symptoms that compound pain, such as nausea, insomnia, and pruritis. |
| Anticonvulsants | Phenytoin, carbamazepine, sodium valproate, clonazepam | Also specific for neuritic pain; helps myoclonic jerks and tics. |
| Skeletal muscle relaxants | Diazepam, clonazepam | Relieves muscle spasm, seizures, anxiety, restlessness, and myoclonus. |
| Smooth muscle relaxants | Belladonna, ditropan | Relieves intestinal cramping and bladder spasms. |
| Butyrophenes | Haloperidol | Relieves anxiety with agitation, nausea, and delirium. |

- Whirlpool

- Exercise/physical therapy

*Psychosocial/spiritual modalities*

- Diversional activities, such as music, art, movies, hobbies, travel, and so forth

- Relaxation and imagery techniques

- Cognitive reframing of control and hopes

- Humor as a stress and pain reliever

- Celebration of normal life events

- Prayer and meditation

- Pastoral visits

- Hypnosis

- Support groups

- Patient education (to address unanswered questions and correct misinformation)

### Drugs to Avoid

Certain drugs are contraindicated for chronic long-term use. They are generally those drugs that have limited effectiveness and undesirable side effects. (See Table 8.6 on the next page.)

## Table 8.6    Drugs to Avoid

| DRUG/DRUG TYPE | RATIONALE |
|---|---|
| Meperidine (Demerol) | Short duration. Repeated doses may lead to central nervous system toxicity. Poor absorption orally. |
| Dronabinol (Marinol) | Too many side effects for routine use (bradycardia, dysphoria, thought impairment, depersonalization). |
| Opioid agonists-antagonists (pentazocine, butorphanol, nalbuphine) | May produce withdrawal symptoms if mixed with opioids, have analgesic ceiling, and may have psychomimetic side effects. |
| Brompton's cocktail | Plain liquid morphine is equally effective without the side effects of the other ingredients as volume of dose is raised. |
| Ketorolac (Toradol) | Recommended only for short-term use due to nephrotoxicity and blood dyscrasias. |
| Placebos | Placebo-derived analgesia may result from endogenous opioids; however, it is short-acting, ultimately ineffective, and destroys patient trust. |
| Cocaine, heroin | No efficacy over available drugs. Illegal in the United States. |

## REFERENCES AND SUGGESTED READINGS

Agency for Health Care Policy and Research. (1995). *Management of cancer pain: Clinical practice guidelines* (Publication No. 94–0592). Rockville, MD: Author.

American Pain Society. (1999). *Principles of analgesic use in the treatment of acute pain and cancer pain* (4th ed.). Skokie, IL: Author.

Ashburn, M. A., & Lipman, A. G. (1993). Management of pain in the cancer patient. *Anesthesia and Analgesia, 76*(2), 402–416.

Bruera, E., Macmillan, K., Pither, J., & MacDonald, R. N. (1990). Effects of morphine on the dyspnea of terminal cancer patients. *Journal of Pain and Symptom Management, 5*(6), 341–344.

Cherny, N. I., & Portenoy, R. K. (1993). Cancer pain management. *Cancer, 72,* 3393–3415.

Cleary, J. F. (1997). Pharmacokinetic and pharmacodynamic issues in the treatment of breakthrough pain. *Seminars in Oncology, 24*(5), 165–195.

Coluzzi, P. H., Volker, B., & Miaskowski, C. (Eds.). (1996). *Comprehensive pain management in terminal illness.* Sacramento: California State Hospice Association.

Cunningham, M. L., Ruger, T. F., & Thorpe, D. M. (Eds.). (1998). *M. D. Anderson Cancer Center nursing reports on strategies for pain management: Assessment of pain syndromes in cancer patients.* Newtown, PA: Associates in Medical Marketing.

Ferrell, B. R., & McCaffery, M. (1997). Nurses' knowledge about equianalgesia and opioid dosing. *Cancer Nursing, 20*(3), 201–212.

Fields, H. L. (1987). *Pain.* New York: McGraw-Hill.

Fields, H. L., & Martin, J. B. (1994). Pain: Pathophysiology and management. In K. J. Isselbacher, E. Braunwald, J. D. Wilson, J. B. Martin, A. S. Fauci, & D. L. Kasper (Eds.), *Harrison's principles of internal medicine* (Suppl. 2). New York: McGraw-Hill.

Foley, K. M. (1993). Pain assessment and cancer pain syndromes. In D. Doyle, G. W. C. Hanks, & N. MacDonald (Eds.), *Oxford textbook of palliative medicine.* Oxford, England: Oxford University Press.

Grond, S., Zech, D., Schugs, S. A., Lynch, J., & Lehman, K. A. (1991).Validation of WHO guidelines for cancer pain—the last days and hours of life. *Journal of Pain and Symptom Management, 6*(7), 411–422.

Hill, C. S., Jr. (1991). *Guidelines for treatment of cancer pain.* Austin: Texas Cancer Council.

Houde, R. W. (1979). Analgesic effectiveness of the narcotic agonist-antagonists. *British Journal of Clinical Pharmacology, 7,* 297S–308S.

Institute of Medicine. (1997). *Approaching death: Improving care at the end of life.* Washington DC: National Academy Press.

Johanson, G. A. (1993). *Physicians' handbook of symptom relief in terminal care* (4th ed.). Santa Rosa: Sonoma County Academic Foundation for Excellence in Medicine.

Kaye, P. (1990). *Notes on symptom control in hospice and palliative care.* Essex, CT: Hospice Education Institute.

Levy, M. H. (1996). Pharmacologic treatment of cancer pain. *New England Journal of Medicine, 335,* 1124–1131.

Melzack, R. (1990). The tragedy of needless pain. *Scientific American, 262*(2), 27–33.

McCaffery, M., & Beebe, A. (1989). *Pain: Clinical manual for nursing practice.* St. Louis: C. V. Mosby.

McCaffery, M., Martin, L., & Ferrell, B. R. (1992). Analgesic administration via rectum or stoma. *ET Nursing, 19*(4), 114–121.

Portenoy, R. K. (1989). Cancer pain: Epidemiology and syndromes. *Cancer, 63,* 2298–2307.

Portenoy, R. K., & Hagen, N. A. (1990). Breakthrough pain: Definition, prevalence, and characteristics. *Pain, 41,* 273–281.

Portenoy, R. K., & Kanner, R. M. (1996). *Pain management: Theory and practice.* Philadelphia: F. A. Davis.

Spross, J. A. (1990). Unrelieved cancer pain: Selections from the literature. *Dimensions of Oncology Nursing, 4*(4), 4–9.

Twycross, R. (1994). *Pain relief in advanced cancer.* New York: Churchill Livingston.

World Health Organization. (1990). *Cancer pain relief and palliative care* (Technical Report Series No. 804). Geneva, Switzerland: Author.

# CHAPTER 9

# Symptom Control

**PURPOSE**

The purpose of this chapter is to describe the principles of appropriate relief of distressing symptoms exhibited by patients who have a terminal illness, toward the goals of excellence in patient comfort and in optimization of quality of life.

**OBJECTIVES**

Upon completion of this chapter, the learner will be able to:

1. List at least three criteria for treatment plan decisions in palliative care

2. Identify two groups of therapeutic measures used in comfort care

3. Discuss the nurse's role in planning for the prevention of recurring symptoms

**CONTENT OUTLINE**

I. Introduction

    A. Goal and focus of palliative care

    B. Criteria for treatment decisions

    C. Consideration of therapeutic response

II. Common Symptoms

    A. Anxiety and insomnia

    B. Confusion, agitation, delirium

    C. Constipation

    D. Cough

  E. Depression

  F. Diarrhea

  G. Dyspnea

  H. Dysphagia

  I. Fluid retention (edema, ascites, pleural effusion)

  J. Hiccups (singultus)

  K. Intestinal obstruction

  L. Nausea and vomiting

  M. Oncologic emergencies

  N. Pruritis

  O. Seizures

  P. Skin problems

  Q. Stomatitis

  R. Terminal airway secretions and restlessness

  S. Urinary problems

  T. Weakness, fatigue, and syncope

# INTRODUCTION

## Goal and Focus of Palliative Care

The goal of palliative care is to apply scientific principles to enhance comfort and quality of life. The focus is relief of distressing symptoms as identified by the patient, which is quite different than intervening in response to an abnormal X-ray or laboratory study. Although the goal and focus are not the same as for acute or curative care, palliative care demands the same application of knowledge from the medical, nursing, psychosocial, nutrition, and pharmacy sciences.

All treatment decisions will depend upon the patient's priorities and the disease trajectory (rapidity of the patient's decline and life expectancy). For example, if it appears evident that the patient has months remaining, the hospice team will suggest different treatment options than when it is obvious the patient has only days or hours.

## Criteria for Treatment Decisions

Leading oncologists have suggested criteria for palliative care decision making that may assist in the transition from acute care to comfort care management. According to Thelma Bates (1987), aggressive treatment is justified in the following circumstances:

- When cure is possible
- When there is a realistic chance of worthwhile prolongation of life
- When the patient chooses a clinical trial with informed consent

The following forms of aggressive treatment are, according to Basil Stoll (1987), inappropriate:

- Aggressive treatment of asymptomatic metastasis
- The use of two or more modalities when one would be adequate
- Prolonged duration of a palliative treatment when the life expectancy is short
- Severe morbidity from a treatment in relation to the degree of hoped-for palliation

Peter Cassileth (Cassileth & Cassileth, 1982) asserts that diagnostic studies should be conducted when the following are true:

- If the results will potentially alter the patient's management
- If the test will help determine the etiology of symptoms before treatment is initiated and its invasiveness does not cause more discomfort than is warranted by the information to be gained
- If the benefits of the results outweigh the physical, emotional, and financial costs of obtaining them
- If the patient's life expectancy is longer than just a few days

To summarize factors involved in decision making, treatment is indicated when these assumptions are reasonable:

- If the outcome is worthwhile (defined by patient comfort), given the trajectory of the illness
- If the potential benefits outweigh the potential risks or burdens to the patient
- If the therapy/test meets the approval of the patient, depending on his or her values, goals, and beliefs
- If the outcome is related to increasing patient comfort, as opposed to battling an unresponsive disease

## Consideration of Therapeutic Response

There is no single "right" way to provide palliative care. Options differ regarding appropriateness or inappropriateness of IVs, surgical
procedures, chemotherapy, or ventilators. It is a challenge to understand the pathophysiology of irreversible end-stage disease, frequently accompanied by multisystems failure, and to realize that
therapeutic value may not be the same as when comparable therapies
are used in acute care with a good chance of response. It is an even
bigger challenge to look honestly at potential outcomes before suggesting a therapy. For example, medication or hydration by clysis
(parenteral injection) is becoming popular, but we need to decide if
we are appeasing our medically oriented mind-set or if such treatment is truly appropriate and beneficial to the patient. Most important, all treatment decisions should be agreeable to the patient and
family, having been made with adequate information about potential
outcomes.

Diagnostic studies are indicated only if they offer information
that will lead to enhanced comfort. Consider a statement made by Dr.
Ira Byock when he was visiting one of his hospice patients, a 46-year-
old man with lung cancer and brain metastases, in the last stages of
his illness: "I realized that he was hallucinating, seeing something on
the patio. I could think of six things that might cause it, but at this
stage these medical musings were of little practical value" (1997, p.
80).

Likewise, vital signs such as temperature, pulse, respiration,
blood pressure, and weight are not routinely taken unless the information gained leads us to improved comfort care. Often vital signs
focus merely on the disease process and the declining condition. For
example, if a patient shows signs of hypotension and is still on antihypertensive medications, it would be worthwhile to obtain repeated
blood pressure readings before discontinuing the medication.
However, if a patient has progressive cachexia and weight loss and
opts not to have artificial feedings, daily weights would serve no useful purpose and in fact would have a negative psychological impact.

The remainder of  this chapter outlines approaches to dealing
with distressing symptoms commonly seen in terminal illness. It is
helpful to hospice team members, as well as community physicians,
if each agency adopts its own set of protocols and standing orders,
building in flexibility for individual physician preferences. Ease of
administration is an important issue to keep in mind as protocols are
developed. For example, if the patient can swallow, oral is always better than parenteral delivery of medication. When the patient cannot
swallow or has trouble swallowing tablets or capsules, it is good to
remember that many drugs now come in liquid form. Further, when

drugs are also available in concentrated liquid form, they can easily be administered sublingually or bucally, even in an unconscious patient.

Nonprescriptive comfort measures are purposely listed first to stimulate consideration of ways to enhance comfort without diagnostic procedures or medical therapies. The former are inexpensive, can be carried out by the family, and do not have to wait for a doctor's order. If nonprescriptive measures work, they are preferable to additional medications or treatments, which have the potential for producing yet more distressing symptoms in the form of side effects.

# Common Symptoms

A word of caution: The following discussion is meant to provide a general overview of these symptoms and palliative measures. All treatments must be chosen on an individual basis and medications prescribed per the pharmaceutical company's current dosing recommendations.

## KEY TO ABBREVIATIONS

| | |
|---|---|
| BID = twice a day | q_h = every _ hours |
| IM = intramuscularly | QID = four times a day |
| IV = intravenously | SC = subcutaneously |
| NPO = nothing by mouth | SL = sublingually |
| PO = by mouth | TID = three times a day |
| PR = rectally | U = units |
| PRN = as needed | |

# Anxiety and Insomnia

Patients with terminal illnesses commonly experience anxiety and/or sleeplessness due to pain, side effects of medications, specific psychosocial concerns, or general fears surrounding terminal illness and death. Sometimes these symptoms are associated with worries about how the family members will manage or how they will endure the moment of death. Patients who use a lot of denial will tend to keep things inside and avoid dialogue about what is happening or what their concerns are.

In milder forms, denial is a useful coping mechanism. The more pronounced the denial, however, the more pronounced the anxiety is apt to be. Hospice team members can allay many fears by openly discussing what symptoms to anticipate and what measures can be taken. Interactions with the patient should make it clear that it is safe to discuss any topic of concern without fear of judgment or repercussion.

## Nonprescriptive Comfort Measures

- Discuss with patient and family whether insomnia is a problem; determine whether the patient is distressed by not sleeping at night or if the family members are getting inadequate rest because of it. Medication is not necessary if sleeplessness is not distressing to anyone involved.

- Talk with, listen to, walk with, and sit by the patient.

- Determine whether fear, pain, or air hunger is present.

- Ask family and volunteers to be present with the patient (if their presence is comforting).

- Decrease stimulation and demands.

- Suggest tub baths or backrubs for relaxation.

- Use music, relaxation tapes, or guided imagery.

- Change the environment according to patient needs (e.g., leave lights on, allow the patient to sleep in a lounge chair).

## Prescriptive Comfort Measures

- For anxiety: Lorazepam (Ativan) 0.5–2 mg PO QID; or diazepam (Valium) 2–10 mg PO, IM, or SL, TID or QID; or alprazolam (Xanax) 0.5–1 mg PO BID, TID, or q6h (alprazolam less desirable because it has no liquid or injectable form and seizures can result from sudden withdrawal).

- For insomnia: Same doses as above at bedtime; or diphenhydramine (Benadryl) 25–50 mg PO at bedtime; or amitriptyline (Elavil) 25–150 mg nightly 1–2 hours before bedtime.

# Confusion, Agitation, Delirium

The symptoms of confusion, agitation, and delirium may all be present at once, present individually, and/or present in varying degrees. Any of these situations is distressing to the patient and the family at a time when they urgently need to be communicating. The causes are so vast and varied that these symptoms are a major challenge to assess. The most likely culprits in terminal illness are side effects of medications, brain metastases, or cerebrovascular accident. Other potential causes include biochemical imbalances; reaction to dementia of neurological conditions; alcohol or drug withdrawal; infection; extreme anxiety; or (especially if the patient cannot communicate) fecal impaction, urinary retention, or pain. (See additional information in the "Terminal Airway Secretions and Restlessness" section of this chapter.)

## Nonprescriptive Comfort Measures

◆ Ascertain patient/family perception of the intensity of symptoms, and assess their values and goals related to proposed interventions.

◆ Speak in a gentle tone to the patient, offering explanations of all events.

◆ Offer the family explanations of causes and stress the importance of ongoing patient orientation.

◆ Explain to the family that it is not unusual for symptoms to exacerbate as night approaches.

◆ Maintain a calm, familiar, and well-lighted environment.

◆ Assess for urinary and bowel problems.

## Prescriptive Comfort Measures

◆ On a trial basis, withhold drugs that may be causing the symptoms, especially in the presence of failing renal or liver function. Drugs with high potential include phenothiazines, benzodiazepines, tricyclics, cimetidine, atropine, beta-blockers, digoxin, pentazocine, and indomethacin.

◆ Give hydroxyzine (Atarax) or lorazepam (Ativan) in low doses for mild agitation and anxiety.

- For confusion or agitation, give lorazepam (Ativan) 1–3 mg PO or SL, BID or TID; or haloperidol (Haldol) 0.5–5 mg PO q6–12h. Give haloperidol 5–10 mg IM for acute agitation.

- Diazepam (Valium) is effective for agitation without psychosis or hallucinations.

- Use tricyclics for agitated depression.

# Constipation

Because terminally ill patients are less active, have diminishing strength and energy, have decreased fluid intake, consume fewer dietary stimulants, and are, generally, on opioids or other drugs that slow the gastrointestinal tract, constipation is a predominant distressing symptom. It is important to remember that patients who are not eating will continue to have some stool and still can become impacted. Constipation can cause new systemic problems, or exacerbate existing ones, including nausea, vomiting, anorexia, pain, or obstruction.

Untreated constipation will result in fecal impaction. This is signified by no bowel movement or by liquid stool seeping around an impaction. For soft impactions, suppositories or enemas may be effective. A hard impaction should be softened first by an oil retention enema, followed by analgesia and/or relaxants prior to manual removal. Most patients are uncomfortable if they go more than 2 or 3 days without a bowel movement, and beyond this impaction may develop quickly.

## Nonprescriptive Comfort Measures

- Ascertain patient/family perception of the intensity of symptoms, and assess their values and goals related to proposed interventions.

- Encourage mobility (pain relief frequently makes this possible).

- Promote fluid intake and dietary stimulants when feasible.

- Provide easy access to toilet or bedside commode and make assistance readily available.

- Obtain a bedside commode if ambulation is a problem (the sitting position facilitates defecation).

- Pursue orders for a bowel stimulant and stool softener when opioids are initiated.

## Prescriptive Comfort Measures

- Order a bowel protocol on every patient who is inactive or on routine opioids.

- Give senna plus docusate sodium (such as Senekot S), 1 cap BID (may increase to 4 caps BID).

- May add milk of magnesia 30 cc with cascara extract 5 ml or lactulose 30–60 cc at bedtime.

- Bisacodyl (Dulcolax) suppository, 10 mg, or Fleets enema can be used to stimulate bowel on third morning or used as the sole agent if the patient cannot swallow.

- Oil retention, soapsuds, or saline enemas may be used to stimulate the bowel.

- Titrate regime to individual patient's need.

# Cough

Persistent, distressful coughing can be caused by the irritation of malignancy, radiation therapy, or infection of chest area; environmental irritants; liquid or solid aspiration; side effects of angio-converting-enzyme (ACE) inhibitors; existing chronic pulmonary disease; bronchospasm; esophageal reflux; pleural effusion; or pulmonary edema.

Unrelieved coughing also can lead to other distresses, such as nausea, vomiting, fatigue from interrupted rest, headaches, or rib fractures if rib metastases are present. A dry cough is harder to manage than a productive cough. Always consider the patient's disease trajectory. For example, you would not give expectorants and mucolytics if the patient is near death and too weak to cough up mucus.

## Nonprescriptive Comfort Measures

- Ascertain patient/family perception of the intensity of symptoms, and assess their values and goals related to proposed interventions.

- Assess for precipitating environmental factors that can be corrected, such as dry air, cool drafts, or cigarette smoke.

- Assist the patient in identifying precipitating factors, such as milk products, cold liquids, and so forth.

- Utilize warm drinks or cough drops to relieve cough.

- Humidify room air if dryness is a problem.

## Prescriptive Comfort Measures

- Use expectorants and mucolytics (terpin hydrate or guaifenesin) for productive cough.

- Give codeine 5–30 mg q4h PRN (dose depends on severity and whether the patient is already on opioids).

- Give morphine sulfate 2–10 mg q4h PRN (dose depends on severity and whether the patient is already on opioids).

- Terminal phase coughing can be relieved with atropine or scopolamine (in the same doses as for terminal secretions).

- Appropriately treat for chronic obstructive pulmonary disease, congestive heart failure, or infections.

- Give benzonatate (Tessalon Perles) 100 mg PO TID for anesthetizing respiratory stretch receptors (only in dry cough).

- Use antireflux medications if this is the etiology of symptoms.

- For severe, unrelieved coughing, nebulized local anesthesia can be used: viscous lidocaine (Xylocaine) 2% for 10 minutes q2–6h (NPO for 30 minutes after treatment).

# Depression

Patients with a terminal illness commonly experience a normal reactive depression. The reactive depression can be a response to diagnosis of a terminal illness, unrelieved symptoms, and/or knowledge of ultimate death. It usually manifests itself in anxieties related to depleted self-esteem, loss of control, frustration and worry about declining physical strength, or physical and emotional impact of the disease. Those patients who tend to hold things inside or feel powerless to take action in the situation may become very withdrawn and are difficult to help.

Normal reactive depression is not the same as clinical endogenous depression. Those with endogenous depression probably have a history of clinical depression, with or without a specific identifiable cause. For known endogenous depression, the usual antidepressants should be initiated.

The approach will be somewhat different with reactive depression. The inappropriate use of antidepressants may lead to unnecessary sedation, dry mouth, worsened constipation, and possible urinary retention. The first-line treatment is psychosocial support from the entire team. This includes having meaningful, unhurried dialogue with the patient to elicit the most overwhelming issues, then responding therapeutically. Such responses may include enhancing physical comfort; having an honest discussion about the future; promoting involvement of family and friends; and giving spiritual comfort, guidance for social and financial problems, and encouragement to "finish business" and conduct life review. Not to be overlooked is the importance of observing usual life events and finding meaningful ways to remain active within physical and emotional constraints. Psychotropic drugs may be given in addition to these measures but are not a substitute.

Because normal reactive depression is an appropriate response to progressive illness and impending death, we should not make it our goal to eradicate the depression but rather should permit patients to evaluate when distress is too great and medication is needed. For example, patients may wish to be medicated if sleeplessness, bad dreams, emotional lability, or persistent deep despair are present and especially distressing.

## Nonprescriptive Comfort Measures

- ◆ Ascertain patient/family perception of the intensity of symptoms, and assess their values and goals related to proposed interventions.

- Establish a trust relationship and follow up by listening fully to what the patient shares.

- Answer the patient's questions honestly in a sensitive and caring, but totally open, manner.

- Involve family, friends, and clergy as indicated.

- Encourage mental and physical activities that may add meaning and satisfaction.

- Do not inhibit tears or outbursts—these may be very therapeutic.

- Help the patient record memories, life review, and important events on audio- or videotape.

- Assure the patient and family of team availability.

## Prescriptive Comfort Measures

- Attend meticulously to symptom control.

- Eliminate potentially offending drugs.

- An anxiolytic drug, along with therapeutic communication, may suffice.

- Give amitriptyline (Elavil) 25–145 mg PO at bedtime. Begin with 25–50 mg and increase by 25–50 mg every 2 to 3 days as tolerated. Amitriptyline is antidepressive/anxiolytic and mildly sedating; it may help the patient sleep when taken in the evening.

- Give doxepin (Sinequan) 50–150 mg PO at bedtime, titrated as described for amitriptyline.

# Diarrhea

Diarrhea is physically exhausting as well as emotionally draining when accidents or odors cause social embarrassment. Only about 5% of terminally ill patients have a problem with diarrhea, and of those the majority are from overflow around fecal impaction, which should be treated with disimpactions, enemas, and an adequate preventive bowel protocol.

Medications causing diarrhea include antibiotics (which destroy normal bowel flora), laxatives used in the treatment of constipation, magnesium-containing antacids, and nonsteroidal anti-inflammatory drugs (NSAIDs). The etiology may also be the disease state, such as in carcinoid tumors, pancreatic cancers, colorectal tumors, or AIDS. Disease treatments such as chemotherapy (which temporarily denudes gastrointestinal epithelium) or radiation (which causes permanent damage to gastrointestinal epithelium) can result in episodic enteritis. Concurrent conditions like ulcerative colitis, irritable bowel syndrome, or opportunistic infections may also be culprits. Lactose intolerance, which often causes diarrhea, may have been a lifelong problem, or it may develop at any point in time.

## Nonprescriptive Comfort Measures

◆ Ascertain patient/family perception of the intensity of symptoms, and assess their values and goals related to proposed interventions.

◆ Suggest avoiding dairy products, using lactose-free milk, or taking lactase tablets (Lactaid) if lactose intolerance suspected.

◆ Reduce dietary fat if the cause is pancreatic insufficiency.

◆ Suggest a dietary consult if the patient concurs.

◆ Protect perianal area with a barrier cream and frequent cleansing.

◆ Note characteristics of stool such as consistency, color, and smell.

◆ Provide easily accessible bathroom or commode to avoid accidents.

◆ Advise the patient that it will be helpful to avoid stimulants such as caffeine or nicotine.

## Prescriptive Comfort Measures

◆ Give loperamide (Imodium) 4 mg tab to start, then 2 mg tab after each loose stool (not to exceed 16 mg/day).

- Give diphenoxylate/atropine (Lomotil) 2 mg PO, then 1 mg after each loose stool, or 1 mg q3–4h PRN (not to exceed 8 mg/day).

- A Fleets enema at a time convenient for the patient allows scheduled evacuation of the lower bowel and decreases the risk of random, unannounced emptying.

- Codeine has a specific side effect of reducing gastrointestinal motility. Dose depends on tolerance and current analgesia (usual dose is 15–30 mg PO q4h).

- Cholestyramine (Questran, Cholybar) 4 g PO, before meals and at bedtime, not to exceed 32 g/day, is indicated if diarrhea is caused by excess bile salts.

- Provide pancreatic enzyme replacement (Pancrease, Viokase, Catozym), 1–3 caps or tabs PO before or with meals if pancreatic enzyme deficiency is suspected.

- Psyllium (Metamucil) is sometimes used because it can absorb fluid from the watery stool.

# Dyspnea

Inability to get sufficient air can be more distressing to the patient and family than pain and is a common symptom in hospice patients. It is seldom the result of a single cause. Multifaceted etiologies may include lung tumors, pleural effusion, congestive heart failure, bronchospasm, or infection. The episodes are almost always exacerbated by anxiety or psychosocial distress. Traditional medical interventions are indicated for conditions that appear reversible, such as digitalis and diuretics for congestive heart failure, or bronchodilators for known chronic obstructive pulmonary disease.

In cases of pneumonitis, in which there is high likelihood of recurrent episodes due to lessening activity, presence of tumor, and poor nutritional status, the decision to give antibiotics depends on disease trajectory and potential for benefit. If rales are present from fluid overload, the patient may benefit from reduced fluid intake. Aspiration of fluid from the chest (thoracentesis) may be considered for severe pleural effusion but does not always change the clinical picture significantly, and fluid can reaccumulate the next day. The use of oxygen is rarely helpful in this population except when associated with restrictive lung disease, and other measures may be of more therapeutic value.

## Nonprescriptive Comfort Measures

- Ascertain patient/family perception of the intensity of symptoms, and assess their values and goals related to proposed interventions.

- Prepare the patient and family by discussing what to expect and actions that might be taken.

- Plan care and activities to decrease exertional dyspnea.

- Position the patient for comfort, sitting upright in bed or chair and/or with arms over a pillow on a table.

- Change the patient's position, with the affected lung down.

- Provide calming and reassurance through the presence of a supportive person.

- Encourage relaxation by using a gentle voice, gentle touching, and guiding slow, deep breaths.

- Keep the room cool and control humidity, depending on patient preferences.

- Move air in the room by fan or by opening a window.

- Solicit the patient's fears and give reassurance about the availability of medications and team members.

## Prescriptive Comfort Measures

- Give morphine sulfate 5 mg SC or SL q3h PRN; may repeat in 20 minutes if necessary. Morphine sulfate reduces inappropriate tachypnea and overventilation of the large airways, making breathing more efficient and without carbon dioxide retention. For the opioid-naive patient, begin with 2.5–5 mg dose.

- Anxiolytics, such as lorazepam (Ativan) 0.5–2 mg q3–6h PRN, can be added to address the anxiety component to dyspnea. Diazepam (Valium) 5–10 mg IM or PO q6h PRN is effective, but it has a longer half-life.

- Bronchodilators, nebulizers, or steroids may be added but generally are helpful only if the patient has a history of these being effective in prior obstructive airway disease.

- Use aerosolized morphine sulfate 4 mg/3–4 cc sodium chloride for panic dyspnea.

- If preceding measures fail, short-acting benzodiazepines can be quickly titrated to a desired level of comfort; sedation may be more desirable than unrelieved dyspnea with high levels of anxiety.

# Dysphagia

Difficult swallowing (dysphagia) or painful swallowing (odynopha-gia) may be directly related to esophageal tumor, radiation-induced stricture, Candida infection, primary head and neck cancers, or external compression from mediastinal metastatic lymph nodes. Some studies have shown that perineural spread of a cancer or pres-sure of tumor or lymph nodes on innervation to the oropharynx can be responsible. Generalized weakness from paraneoplastic syn-dromes, end-stage debilitating disease, or neuromuscular disorders can all lead to dysphagia. Skull, meningeal, or cerebral infiltration by tumor can result in cranial nerve (or bulbar) palsy, leading to dis-abled swallowing mechanisms.

## Nonprescriptive Comfort Measures

- Ascertain patient/family perception of the intensity of symptoms, and assess their values and goals related to proposed interven-tions.

- Elevate the patient's head during meals and for 30 minutes after-ward.

- Tipping the chin slightly downward will decrease likelihood of aspiration in most patients.

- Pay close attention to good oral hygiene.

- Work with the patient and family to determine the consistency of food best tolerated. It is assumed liquids or soft foods are prefer-able, but this is not always the case.

## Prescriptive Comfort Measures

- Use viscous lidocaine (Xylocaine) 2%, 1–2 teaspoons to swish and swallow q3h PRN for pain. (Caution patient and family about difficulty swallowing if tongue and throat are numb.)

- Use nystatin suspension (Mycostatin) 600,000 U QID for *Candida esophagitis.*

- Give ketoconazole (Nizoral) 200–400 mg PO daily if nystatin is not effective.

- Dexamethasone (Decadron) 8–12 mg/day may offer temporary relief by reducing inflammatory edema, but after a few weeks myopathy and other steroid side effects may develop.

♦ More aggressive measures such as bypass surgery, laser treatment, or endoprosthetic intubation are rarely good options due to high probability of serious complications. The symptom itself portends limited prognosis.

# Fluid Retention: Edema, Ascites, Pleural Effusion

Patients with irreversible end-stage illnesses frequently develop extracellular fluid retention, such as edema, ascites, and pleural effusion. These can result from malignant cell activity, lymphadenopathy, congestive heart failure, immobility, renal failure, protein deficiency, or medications causing fluid retention, such as steroids or NSAIDs.

As mentioned in the section on dyspnea, few of the invasive procedures result in any significant or long-lasting improvement. In select cases, a thoracentesis, paracentesis, or Leveen shunt may be beneficial, but the mainstays of management are diuretics and avoidance of overhydration.

Improving the nutritional status to eliminate protein deficiency would help but may not be feasible or appropriate for most of these patients. Tumor edema, especially in the brain or gastrointestinal tract, may be alleviated temporarily by a steroid regimen.

In most patients the manifestation of systemic edema is determined by gravity (e.g., in the lower extremities when the patient is up or sitting most of the time, or in the back when the patient spends most of the time in bed). This is generally referred to as *dependent edema*.

## Nonprescriptive Comfort Measures

+ Ascertain patient/family perception of the intensity of symptoms, and assess their values and goals related to proposed interventions.

+ Encourage exercise, especially leg exercises, even if the patient is bed bound.

+ Leg elevation helps but only when legs are level with the right atrium of the heart. For this reason, it is seldom useful to elevate legs while the patient is sitting in a chair.

+ Encourage increase in dietary protein in cases where the patient is able and willing.

## Prescriptive Comfort Measures

+ Use compression stockings (thigh-high) for daytime out-of-bed hours.

◆ Cautiously use oral diuretics, such as hydrochlorothiazide in a moderate dose three times a week as a trial (recognizing distresses associated with diuresis and symptoms of electrolyte imbalance).

◆ For severe ascites: Give spironolactone 200 mg plus furosemide 40 mg daily; continue up to 4 weeks if it is beneficial.

◆ Medicate for pain and/or dyspnea.

# Hiccups (Singultus)

Prolonged hiccups, lasting hours or days, can be physically and emotionally exhausting. The etiology is stress to the diaphragm, which may be chemical (infections, pancreatitis, uremia), mechanical (pressure or local extension of tumor, gastric distention, hepatomegaly), or neurological (phrenic nerve or vagus nerve irritation, brain-stem tumors). Phrenic nerve block does not guarantee relief and is rarely considered.

## Nonprescriptive Comfort Measures

♦ Ascertain patient/family perception of the intensity of symptoms, and assess their values and goals related to proposed interventions.

♦ Suggest pharyngeal stimulation by means such as the following:

Swallowing 2 teaspoons of sugar

Drinking ice water or swallowing crushed ice

Using a rebreathing bag or mask

Holding the breath

Massaging midline of soft palate for 1 minute with a toothette or cotton swab

## Prescriptive Comfort Measures

♦ Use any of the following:

Simethicone (in Mylanta, Mylicon, Maalox Plus) if gastric distention is present

Chlorpromazine (Thorazine) 25 mg PO or PR TID

Metoclopromide (Reglan) 10–20 mg PO after meals and at bedtime

Diazepam (Valium) 5–10 mg PO q4–6h

Prednisone 5 mg PO daily if hepatomegaly or tumor invasion exists. Maximum dose is 60 mg/day and should be tapered when symptoms are relieved or if the medication is not helping.

Baclofen (Lioresal) 5 mg TID

Nifedipine (Procardia) 10 mg TID (consider whether it is worth the side effects)

- Teach the patient and family about the potential for hypotension with use of diazepam (Valium), baclofen (Lioresal), or chlorpromazine (Thorazine).

# Intestinal Obstruction

This serious symptom should be managed only after taking into consideration the cause and level of obstruction, how large a tumor mass may be, presence of multiple compressing lesions, the general condition of the patient, and the expected disease trajectory. Surgery has traditionally been the primary treatment for intestinal obstruction, but it is now recognized that patients with advanced and widespread disease and who are in poor general condition probably will not benefit, even if they survive the surgery. One surgical consultant at St. Christopher's Hospice gave as his criteria for surgery: "Good evidence of a single block in a relatively fit patient." Unfortunately, the results of palliative surgery are not good, measured both by mean survival time and symptom control. There is a high surgical mortality, high rate of re-obstruction, and poor relief of symptoms. For the majority in terminal phases of disease, it is more beneficial to utilize conservative comfort measures and symptom management, including medication for colicky pain, nausea, and vomiting. Some patients will choose the option of a nasogastric tube for suction, whereas a few may choose to ingest food and fluids, knowing they will vomit, instead of suffering the discomfort of the nasogastric tube. If the patient is not given IV fluids, the resulting dehydration sometimes relieves the obstruction.

## Nonprescriptive Comfort Measures

+ Ascertain patient/family perception of the intensity of symptoms, and assess their values and goals related to proposed interventions.

+ Evaluate for possible impaction.

+ Assess patterns of obstruction (those with intermittent symptoms may have spontaneous return of bowel function).

+ Offer ice chips for dry mouth.

## Prescriptive Comfort Measures

+ Perform a rectal exam to rule out impaction.

+ Consider surgical resection if there is a single removable blocking mass and no large abdominal tumor masses, and the patient is in good physical condition and wishes to have surgery.

- Use scopolamine for colicky pain (0.8–2.4 mg per 24 hours).

- Use narcotics for visceral pain.

- Use haloperidol (Haldol) for nausea (5–10 mg per 24 hours), SC or PR.

- Patients should be allowed to eat and drink as they choose.

# Nausea and Vomiting

The causes of nausea and vomiting are varied, and these symptoms usually have a high anxiety component. Assessment must include possible contributing etiologies such as drugs (especially NSAIDs, aspirin, potassium, theophylline toxicity, digitalis toxicity, or analgesics), pain, constipation/obstruction, esophageal lesion or infection, hepatic failure, azotemia, increased intracranial pressure, peptic ulcer, poor gastric emptying, or psychogenic causes. Antiemetics should be used immediately to give relief while determining the etiology. If symptoms are side effects of a particular medication, use a substitute when possible; if not, give an antiemetic with or prior to each dose. Projectile vomiting may be due to obstruction or increased intracranial pressure. Brain tumors will frequently but not indefinitely respond to steroid therapy. Communication with the patient can determine whether noxious smells, anxieties, or fears are factors.

## Nonprescriptive Comfort Measures

+ Ascertain patient/family perception of the intensity of symptoms, and assess their values and goals related to proposed interventions.

+ Remind the patient that nausea from opioids usually subsides after the initial 2 to 3 days.

+ Activities that may relax and distract the patient are beneficial to treat the psychological component.

+ Assess the patient for relationship of nausea to particular medications or other significant patterns.

+ Allow the patient to self-regulate intake, suggesting decrease in fatty, gas forming, or fried foods.

+ Eliminate strong or repulsive odors.

+ Offer small, frequent meals and, especially, cold foods with minimal odors.

+ Provide a restful environment; ascertain and deal with anxieties.

## Prescriptive Comfort Measures

+ Discontinue offending medications when possible.

+ Use prochlorperazine (Compazine) 10 mg PO or IM q4h PRN, or 25 mg rectally q12h PRN.

- If symptoms derive from liver failure, consider a trial of lactulose (Cephulac) 30 cc TID adjusted to achieve two to three soft stools per day.

- Alprazolam (Xanax) 0.5 mg PO q6h PRN has both an antianxiety and antiemetic effect.

- Use metoclopramide (Reglan) 10 mg PO or IM q6h PRN, or before meals and at bedtime.

- If gastric irritation is from medication or known peptic ulcer disease, an $H_2$ receptor antagonist will help: Cimetidine (Tagamet), ranitidine (Zantac), or famotidine (Pepcid).

- Give haloperidol (Haldol) 0.5–2.0 mg PO or SC q6h PRN. This is a useful drug because it is a strong antiemetic causing low sedation. It has less anticholinergic effect and fewer cardiac and central nervous system side effects, as compared to phenothiazines. It is also long acting, economical, and comes in liquid and injectable form. Routine use of 1–1.5 mg at bedtime for 3 to 4 days after initiating opioids may avert nausea.

- Ondansetron (Zofran) is rarely useful in this population.

# Oncologic Emergencies

*Emergency* connotes sudden onset of life-threatening symptoms, to which we usually respond with rapid and intensive therapies. However, this is not an appropriate response when the patient's condition and prognosis are such that the usual intensive therapies would be futile for cure, improvement, or comfort. In palliative care for terminal illness, it is wise to anticipate crisis events and preplan the actions that will be taken. Decisions should take into consideration any potential benefit to the patient, the disease trajectory, and the patient's goals. Following are some of the choices of management for palliative/comfort care in emergencies associated with advanced terminal illness.

## Hemorrhage

Hemorrhage most often occurs as a result of a tumor's eroding into a major blood vessel. External hemorrhage can be very traumatic to the patient and others present; this happens most often with head and neck or lung cancers. Prepare the family for this potential, have dark towels or blankets available to absorb the blood, and have PRN sedative medications on order for calming the patient. Erosion by tumor with resultant hemorrhage can occur anywhere in the body and frequently is the terminal event. Serious but more prolonged bleeding can occur in the bladder, and continuous irrigation may be needed for comfort (to prevent clots from accumulating). Warfarin (Coumadin) should be discontinued in the terminal phase of illness.

## Hypercalcemia

Hypercalcemia is common in patients with extensive bone metastases, especially in breast and lung cancers. It may present as drowsiness, nausea, confusion, and muscle weakness, but these symptoms are frequently already present in end-stage disease, so it may be hard to distinguish. Pamidronate (Aredia) given intravenously is the treatment of choice but would be used only if the patient concurs that the temporary improvement is worth the IV, labs, and other inconveniences. Much depends on the disease trajectory. Immobility and dehydration increase the chances of the development or recurrence of hypercalcemia, and they are both usually present in end-stage disease.

## Spinal cord compression

Spinal cord compression usually presents in terminal conditions as a result of tumor or collapsed vertebrae from bone metastases, which exert pressure on the spinal cord. This condition requires treatment within 24 to 48 hours by radiation therapy to prevent paralysis. Caregivers must recognize and immediately report symptoms of back pain, weakness or numbness of the legs, or urinary hesitancy or retention. Dexamethasone (Decadron) is usually given immediately. An indwelling catheter and analgesics will provide comfort.

### Superior vena cava syndrome

Superior vena cava syndrome is obstruction of blood flow in this major vessel by the pressure of a tumor or enlarged nodes in the upper chest. The patient may have facial, neck, and arm edema; dyspnea; and development of collateral circulation (i.e., dilated, small veins on chest, arms, and neck). The patient also may have hoarseness, dysphagia, or stridor if these masses press on larynx, esophagus, or laryngeal nerves. The usual treatment is dexamethasone (Decadron) and radiation therapy. For a responsive cancer such as lymphoma or small-cell cancer of the lung, chemotherapy will be equally effective. Opioids and anxiolytics will provide comfort.

# Pruritis

In patients with a terminal illness, pruritis occurs most often because of cholestasis (biliary obstruction), which results in bile salt retention in the skin, with or without obvious jaundice. The usual cause is liver metastases, but pruritis also occurs with liver or gallbladder primary cancer. It can also be caused by an allergic reaction, in which case a rash also may be present and the patient will get relief from antihistamines. Itching increases in intensity with overheating, anxiety, boredom, and dry skin.

## Nonprescriptive Comfort Measures

♦ Ascertain patient/family perception of the intensity of symptoms, and assess their values and goals related to proposed interventions.

♦ Apply emollient lotions to moisten the skin; the gentle rubbing action also gives temporary relief.

♦ Keep room temperatures comfortably cool.

♦ Provide cool starch baths (hot baths will exacerbate itching).

## Prescriptive Comfort Measures

♦ Promethazine (Phenergan) 25–50 mg PO at bedtime may give relief from itching and enhance sleep.

♦ Apply calamine lotion to the skin.

♦ Use steroid skin creams if itching is severe and unresponsive to other therapy.

♦ Use hydroxyzine (Atarax) 25–50 mg PO q8h or diphenhydramine (Benadryl) 25–50 mg PO q6h PRN.

♦ Cholestyramine (Questran, Cholybar) 4 gm PO before meals and at bedtime, not to exceed 32 g/day, may be given a trial if pruritis is associated with biliary obstruction.

♦ High-dose steroids may temporarily relieve biliary pressure.

# Seizures

Seizures do not occur frequently in terminally ill patients, but seizure activity is such a traumatic event that even the unconscious patient should be treated to lessen the duration and prevent recurrence. Once a patient experiences focal or full-blown seizures, anticonvulsive therapy should be given prophylactically. In the event of recurrent seizures, a PRN order of diazepam (Valium) should be routinely ordered in addition to daily orders of anticonvulsants.

The most probable cause of seizures is brain tumor, primary or metastatic. Less likely are seizures from cerebrovascular accident, abscess, increased intracranial pressure, uremia, medications, or hyponatremia.

## Nonprescriptive Comfort Measures

- ◆ Ascertain patient/family perception of the intensity of symptoms, and assess their values and goals related to proposed interventions.

- ◆ Talk with the patient and/or family about seizure activity; it is usually a frightening thing to experience.

- ◆ Gently protect the patient from falls or injury during the seizure; protect the tongue by inserting padded tongue blades between the teeth.

- ◆ Never forcefully restrain movement or a rigid extremity.

- ◆ Do not leave the patient alone during or immediately following a seizure.

- ◆ Following seizure, the patient should be covered with a blanket and allowed to rest.

- ◆ Do not give food, liquids, or oral medicines until the patient is fully alert; the postictal period can last for varying periods of time.

- ◆ Patients prone to seizures will benefit from a calm atmosphere with low levels of noise, confusion, and bright lights.

## Prescriptive Comfort Measures

- ◆ Use diazepam (Valium) 10 mg IM for seizure, with repeated doses if necessary. Following the seizure, routine anticonvulsive therapy should be started. Phenytoin (Dilantin) 300 mg PO at bedtime is usually the drug of choice. An alternative is valproate (Depakene) 200 mg PO TID.

- ◆ For focal seizure prevention, use carbamazepine (Tegretol) 200 mg PO BID.

- ◆ IM phenobarbitol or SL lorazepam (Ativan) or diazepam (Valium) may be used when the patient is unconscious or cannot swallow.

# Skin Problems

Due to poor nutritional status and increasing immobility, all terminal patients are at risk for pressure ulcers. These most frequently occur over bony prominences and weight-bearing areas, most commonly the hips, sacrum, and heels. How rapidly pressure ulcers develop varies with each patient, but the risk can be decreased with aggressive measures to relieve pressure on vulnerable areas and improve circulation, and by keeping bedsheets smooth, dry, and clean. The key to care of pressure ulcers is to remember that they are easier to prevent than to treat. Draining wounds, fistulas, and fungating lesions cannot always be prevented, but measures can be taken to minimize the extent of surrounding skin breakdown. The ostomy nurse can usually be of assistance in assessment and treatment planning. The general goal is to keep an open wound moist, while keeping intact skin clean and dry.

## Nonprescriptive Comfort Measures

- Ascertain patient/family perception of the intensity of symptoms, and assess their values and goals related to proposed interventions.

- Maintain good position and body alignment.

- Turn the patient at least every 2 hours.

- Keep local area dry, clean, and free of body wastes.

- Use pressure-releasing devices such as pillows, pads, and special mattresses.

- In repositioning the patient in bed or transferring the patient, use techniques that reduce friction or pressure. Allowing a reddened area (Stage I) to rub against sheets can cause a blister or break the skin (Stage II).

- Encourage as much mobility as possible.

## Prescriptive Comfort Measures

- For Stage I (redness): Use creams, ointments, or sprays.

- For Stage II (blister or break in the skin): Use a semipermeable dressing (e.g., bioclusives or hydrocolloidal dressings such as Duoderm) if no infection is present.

+ For Stage III (destruction of subcutaneous tissue): Use surgical debridement, wet-to-dry saline dressings, hydrocolloidal dressings, antimicrobials, hydrogen peroxide, or whirlpool therapy.

+ For Stage IV (muscle or bone involvement): Use wet-to-dry dressings; surgical debridement may be needed depending on disease trajectory.

+ For skin and wound infections, use appropriate oral or topical antibiotics.

# Stomatitis

Inflamed oral mucosa can be very uncomfortable and severe enough to preclude eating. If there is concomitant xerostomia, or lack of saliva, the condition will worsen, and ultimately a superimposed infection will occur (most commonly *Candida*). It is important to keep in mind that a *Candida* infection of the oral cavity often extends into the esophagus and can result in additional symptoms, such as nausea and dysphagia. The propensity for infection is directly related to the degree of immunosuppression.

Chemotherapy can cause a temporary denuding of the mucosal epithelium, resulting in oral mucositis. Radiation therapy can result in longer lasting tissue destruction, plus chronic or permanent damage to the saliva glands, depending on the radiation field. Other causes are drug side effects (especially of antibiotics and steroids), fever, dehydration, and dryness from oxygen therapy.

## Nonprescriptive Comfort Measures

- Ascertain patient/family perception of the intensity of symptoms, and assess their values and goals related to proposed interventions.

- Establish a preventive oral hygiene protocol in patients at risk.

- Maintain oral hygiene through frequent but gentle use of a soft toothbrush, toothette, or wet gauze.

- Avoid alcohol-based mouthwashes and cleaning solutions such as glycerin swabs.

- Offer frozen pops made of fruit juice or tonic water.

- For dry mouth, suggest frequent sips of liquids.

- Advise the patient to avoid very hot foods, spicy items, or acidic juices.

- Check dentures to determine whether they need relining to fit properly and to prevent abrasion of tissues.

- Cleanse dentures frequently and soak in diluted bleach (1 part sodium hypochlorite to 80 parts water).

## Prescriptive Comfort Measures

- Use Xerolube (or other artificial saliva), 5 cc orally as often as desired.

- Nystatin (Mycostatin) oral suspension, 100,000 units; swish and swallow QID for fungal infection.

- Use ketoconazole (Nizoral) PO 200–400 mg daily; stop when thrush is cleared up.

- Use clotrimazole (Mycelex), dissolve one lozenge in mouth 5 times a day for 2 weeks.

- Fluconazole (Diflucan) PO or IV may be used for unresponsive and distressing fungal disease.

- Viscous lidocaine (Xylocaine) 2%; swish and swallow 10 cc q3h PRN for comfort.

- Solution of equal parts antacid solution (Mylanta), diphenhydramine (Benadryl) elixir, and viscous lidocaine (Xylocaine) 2%; swish and swallow 10 cc q3h PRN for comfort.

# Terminal Airway Secretions and Restlessness

Terminal airway secretions accumulate when the patient is stuperous and unable to swallow saliva and has upper-respiratory tract secretions or fluid overload that cannot be coughed up. These deep, moist, noisy respirations associated with an ineffective, nonproductive cough are commonly referred to as the "death rattle." This is a common occurrence in the last 12 to 24 hours of life. The patient is usually oblivious to this phenomenon, but it is distressing to loved ones. In some cases, suctioning the patient may be necessary for the sake of the family.

Some patients will also experience moderate to severe terminal agitation and/or restlessness. If they are beyond communicating, sedatives are appropriate to relieve these symptoms.

Family members may need to be given permission to take a break from a bedside watch. Some will be reassured that taking a break is OK if they know someone else will be present with the patient. Others may have the need to remain at the bedside until the end.

## Nonprescriptive Comfort Measures

- Ascertain patient/family perception of the intensity of symptoms, and assess their values and goals related to proposed interventions.

- Support family members and remind them that touching and speaking to the patient may be very comforting.

- Allow family members to be involved in care if they wish; this can be therapeutic for them.

- Provide frequent mouth care, especially if the patient is open-mouth breathing.

- Instill artificial tears if the patient's eyes are open and drying out.

- To clear airway, turn the patient on his or her side and change position every 2 hours unless the patient seems bothered by this.

- Remind the family not to push fluids, as this will increase the bothersome secretions.

- Reassure the family that the patient will be made comfortable during this expected final stage.

- Check the patient's bladder for retention (highly likely if anticholinergic drugs are used).

- Consider pain as a cause for agitation, especially if the patient has a known pain syndrome.

## Prescriptive Comfort Measures

- Give morphine sulfate 5 mg SL, bucally, or SC q4h PRN for restlessness, dyspnea, or pain.

- Use the scopolamine patch for the anticholinergic effect of reducing secretions, or scopolamine or atropine 0.4–1.0 mg SC or IM q4h PRN (scopolamine is more sedating).

- Continue whatever analgesic doses the patient has been on; untreated pain can cause an agonal end, and stopping an opioid suddenly can cause the patient to suffer withdrawal symptoms.

- Diazepam (Valium) 5–20 mg is helpful, especially if twitching or focal seizures are present; also useful is lorazepam (Ativan) 1–2 mg.

- Give chlorpromazine (Thorazine) 25–75 mg IM q4h for restlessness.

- Midazolam (Versed) is a rapid and short-acting sedative as well as being effective for seizures, anxiety, dyspnea, and muscle spasm.

- Other effective sedatives include phenobarbital, methotrimeprazine (Levoprome), droperidol (Inapsine), and haloperidol (Haldol).

# Urinary Problems

Urinary retention or incontinence may be related to the terminal condition, as in dysfunctional innervation in end-stage multiple sclerosis, cancer resulting in obstructive tumor pressure, fistulas, or spinal cord compression. In older patients, these problems often result from natural physiological deterioration (e.g., sphincter or muscle weakness), a treatable episodic condition such as infection or constipation, or side effects of medications. In elderly men, varying degrees of obstruction may be present due to benign prostatic hypertrophy. For many chronically ill or elderly patients, the problem may be impaired awareness or inability to communicate.

Anticholinergic medications such as antihistamines, phenothiazines, and tricyclics may cause hesitancy or retention. Sedative drugs tend to increase nighttime incontinence. Diuretics may result in excessive output that is not manageable by the debilitated patient. Recurring chronic cystitis may be secondary to previous chemotherapy treatment with cyclophosphamide (Cytoxan) or the result of radiation therapy. Medications commonly prescribed for bladder problems should be used cautiously because they can cause unwanted side effects. For example, anticholinergics may be used as a bladder relaxant but can lead to hesitancy and retention.

The challenge is to identify and take action to correct reversible conditions, such as infection or bowel impaction. When this is not possible, comfort should be individualized for each patient. For example, one patient/family may prefer frequent changes and increased laundering as opposed to dealing with a catheter, whereas another would prefer the catheter and its attendant problems.

## Nonprescriptive Comfort Measures

♦ Ascertain patient/family perception of the intensity of symptoms, and assess their values and goals related to proposed interventions.

♦ For patients with dysphasia, restlessness frequently indicates the need to void.

♦ Use linens or disposable pads to absorb urine.

♦ Provide frequent skin care, keeping skin clean and dry, and protecting it with petroleum jelly or other moisture barriers.

♦ Retention may be relieved by the sound of running water, warm compresses to the perineum, sitting in a tub, or standing in a shower.

- Suggest increased fluid intake to decrease infections (especially acidic juices such as cranberry).

- For the patient who is confused or needs assistance ambulating, facilitate periodic trips to the toilet or commode chair as a preventive measure.

- Palpate the bladder to ascertain if incontinence is actually retention with overflow.

- Review history of bowel and bladder habits and examine rectum, if indicated, to rule out impacted bowel as a cause of retention.

- Review medications for potential beneficial changes.

## Prescriptive Comfort Measures

- Catheterization may provide relief of uncomfortable retention.

- An indwelling urinary catheter can be employed when incontinence is a problem and external drains not tolerated.

- The following also may be useful:

    Bethanechol (Urecholine) PO 10–50 mg BID to QID if the problem is poor bladder contraction

    Trimethoprim-sulfamethoxazole (TMP-SMZ, Bactrim, Septra) PO 160 mg TMP/800 mg SMX, q12h for 10 to 14 days for symptomatic infection. (Sometimes continued as prophylaxis.)

    Flavoxate (Urispas) 100–200 mg PO TID to QID for bladder spasms

    Oxybutynin (Ditropan) PO 5 mg BID to QID for bladder spasms

    Imipramine (Tofranil) PO 10–25 mg TID for bladder spasms

    B & O suppositories q3h PRN for painful bladder spasms

    Desmopressin acetate (Concentraid, DDAVP), IV, SC, or nasal spray for nocturnal enuresis

# Weakness, Fatigue, and Syncope

All three of these symptoms are common in chronic progressive disease. Fatigue is actually one of the diagnostic features of cancer and other diseases and worsens as patients go through treatments and the disease progresses. Weakness is usually progressive with concomitant weight loss, decreased mobility, and declining performance status. Declining functional status, as measured by the Karnofsky Performance Status Scale or increased dependence in activities of daily living, is indicative of a poor prognosis. Syncope (temporary suspension of respiration and circulation) usually comes at a later stage, with decreased muscle tone and hypotension. It is important to monitor blood pressure if the patient is on antihypertensive drugs to ascertain when these may no longer be indicated.

Dr. Peter Kaye (1990) states, "There is no drug that restores strength" (p. 311). Because there is no cure for these symptoms, the focus should be on optimizing safety and whatever potential the patient has for desired activity.

## Nonprescriptive Comfort Measures

♦ Ascertain patient/family perception of the intensity of symptoms, and assess their values and goals related to proposed interventions.

♦ Physical therapy may be possible once the patient is relieved of other symptoms, such as pain.

♦ An electric bed, walker, handrails, or raised toilet seat may increase independence.

♦ Permit the patient to function as independently as desired, even though tasks may take much more time and be less efficient.

♦ Assist the patient in listing priorities and planning to conserve energy for special events and desired activities.

♦ Teach the patient and family the importance of gradual position changes from lying to sitting to standing prior to ambulation.

♦ Daily passive range-of-motion exercises may be useful in slowing the progress of disability, if agreed upon by patient/family and therapist.

♦ Planning an activity desired by, and appealing to, the patient may address the patient's psychosocial needs and lessen depression.

## Prescriptive Comfort Measures

- Discontinue any unnecessary antihypertensives.

- Evaluate for hypokalemia if the patient has been on diuretics or has had persistent vomiting or diarrhea.

- Dexamethasone (Decadron) PO 4 mg/day may give a sense of well-being, but the patient should be informed that the effect may be temporary.

## References and Suggested Readings

Amenta, M. O., & Bohnet, N. L. (1986). *Nursing care of the terminally ill.* Boston: Little, Brown.

Bates, T. D. (Ed.). (1987). *Ballière's clinical oncology: International practice and research: Vol. 1/No. 2. Contemporary palliation of difficult symptoms.* London: Tindall.

Byock, I. R. (1997). *Dying well: The prospect for growth at the end of life.* New York: Riverhead Books.

Cassileth, B. R., & Cassileth, P. A. (1982). *Clinical care of the terminal cancer patient.* Philadelphia: Lea & Febiger.

Doyle, D. (Ed.). (1984). *Palliative care: The management of far advanced illness.* Philadelphia: Charles.

Doyle, D., Hanks, G. W. C., & MacDonald, N. (Eds.). (1998). *Oxford textbook of palliative medicine* (2nd ed.). New York: Oxford University Press.

Enck, R. E. (1994). *The medical care of terminally ill patients.* Baltimore: Johns Hopkins University Press.

Hull, R. A. (1994). *Pocketbook of palliative care.* New York: McGraw-Hill.

Johanson, G. A. (1993). *Physicians' handbook of symptom relief in terminal care* (4th ed.). Santa Rosa: Sonoma County Academic Foundation for Excellence in Medicine.

Kaye, P. (1990). *Notes on symptom control in hospice and palliative care.* Essex, CT: Hospice Education Institute.

Kemp, C. (1999). *Terminal illness: A guide to nursing care* (2nd ed.). Philadelphia: J. B. Lippincott.

Levy, M. H. (1985). Pain management in advanced cancer. *Seminars in Oncology, 12*(4), 394–410.

Levy, M. H., & Catalano, R. B. (1985). Control of common physical symptoms other than pain in patients with terminal disease. *Seminars in Oncology, 12*(4), 411–430.

Saunders, C., Baines, M., & Dunlop, K. (1995). *Living with dying: A guide to palliative care* (3rd ed.). New York: Oxford University Press.

Sheehan, D. C., & Forman, W. (1996). *Hospice and palliative care.* Boston: Jones and Bartlett.

Stoll, B. A. (1987). Knowing when not to treat. In T. D. Bates (Ed.), *Ballière's clinical oncology: International practice and research: Vol. 1/No.2. Contemporary palliation of difficult symptoms.* London: Tindall.

Storey, P. (1994). *Primer of palliative care.* Gainesville, FL: Academy of Hospice Physicians.

Storey, P., & Knight, C. F. (1996). *Management of selected nonpain symptoms in the terminally ill.* Gainesville, FL: American Academy of Hospice and Palliative Medicine.

Wrede-Seaman, L. (1999). *Symptom management algorithms: A handbook for palliative care* (2nd ed.). Yakima, WA: Intellicard.

Zimmerman, J. M. (1986). *Complete care for the terminally ill* (2nd ed.). Baltimore: Urban and Schwarzenberg.

# CHAPTER 10

# Palliative Nutrition and Hydration

## PURPOSE

The purpose of this chapter is to review the benefits and burdens of artificially provided nutrition and hydration in end-stage terminal illness and to present the idea that research as well as professional and legal opinions support a conservative approach.

## OBJECTIVES

Upon completion of this chapter, the learner will be able to:

1. Define palliative nutrition and hydration
2. List some content items to include in family teaching on the subject
3. Discuss the moral, medical, and ethical issues surrounding provision of artificial nutrition and hydration in terminal stages
4. Relate research findings to comfort and longevity in dehydrated dying patients

## CONTENT OUTLINE

I. Defining Palliative Nutrition and Hydration

    A. Satisfying patient desires

    B. Optimizing intake and comfort

    C. Relieving symptoms with parenteral hydration

II. Family Teaching

    A. Understanding nutritional needs

    B. Refocusing caring emotions

III. The Dilemma of Artificial Nutrition and Hydration in Terminal Illness

    A.  Morality of caring

    B.  Medical imperatives

    C.  Ethical and legal concerns

IV. Nutrition and Hydration Benefits and Burdens

    A.  Relationship to comfort

    B.  Relationship to distressing complications

    C.  Relationship to longevity

# DEFINING PALLIATIVE NUTRITION AND HYDRATION

## Satisfying Patient Desires

The primary goal of nutrition and hydration in terminal illness is patient comfort. The traditional goal of nutritional repletion, or the achievement of ideal weight with metabolic balance, is neither realistic nor appropriate in progressive end-stage disease. Therefore, palliative nutrition translates to a diet the patient tolerates and desires, on demand. Restricted diets are rarely necessary. The diet should be restricted only if the patient prefers. Some patients who have been restricted in sodium in the past are accustomed to and prefer the taste of food cooked without salt; diabetics may prefer not to consume sugar-laden foods. However, it is common for a patient with end-stage cancer to prefer sweets to proteins and fats. Untoward side effects rarely occur because total intake is so diminished that the amount of sodium, sugar, cholesterol, and calories is self-limited.

## Optimizing Intake and Comfort

Patients who are seriously ill have early satiety—meaning they cannot eat very much without feeling full or satisfied. Offering small but more frequent feedings will optimize intake and result in increased comfort. Following are some additional suggestions to achieve these same goals:

- Encourage high-protein/high-calorie foods, such as eggs, milkshakes, custards, peanut butter, and cream soups.

- Powdered nutritional supplements can be added to other foods without adding volume.

- Do not force foods that cause a metallic or bitter taste. These are usually red meats; fish or poultry could be offered instead.

- If an aversion to all meats develops, try eggs, cheese, or beans for protein.

- Provide food whenever the patient expresses hunger; do not wait for mealtime or expect the patient to eat three meals a day.

- Encourage intake gently, without pressure.

- Remove food when the patient is finished.

- Offer favorite foods; expect changes from previous preferences.

- Make the atmosphere and food presentation as pleasant as possible.

- To conserve energy and/or reduce frustration, use "sippy cups" or large straws.

- Steroids may stimulate appetite; discontinue if side effects outweigh benefits.

- Megesterol acetate (Megace) in doses of 800 mg per day may increase appetite but can be costly.

- Beer, wine, or sherry before meals may help appetite.

- Have ill-fitting dentures relined if this is a problem.

- Avoid routine weighing; it places undue emphasis on weight loss.

Patients who are on tube feedings need special attention to optimize benefits while minimizing complications. The most common and serious complication of tube feedings is aspiration into the lungs. Aspiration may be due to stomach overloading, vomiting, poor sphincter control, or tube migration. Because we cannot assume the metabolism and absorption of fluids and nutrients in terminally ill patients will be normal, frequent testing of residual in the stomach is necessary. This will help determine the amount and frequency of feeding possible without overloading. It will also help in decisions about bolus versus continuous drip methods of feeding. Elevation of the head for 1 hour after a bolus feeding is helpful. Other complications to be aware of are erosion and inflammation of the tissues around the tubing. With long-term use of nasogastric tubes, nasal or esophageal necrosis can occur. With gastrostomies or jejunostomies, the ostomy opening must be kept clean and dry to prevent erosion and irritation.

Permitting the patient to be in control (i.e., deciding the quantity, quality, and frequency) is the best way to maximize intake while minimizing discomfort. The hospice team can be of assistance in three ways: (a) establishing the patient's wishes, (b) planning interventions and ameliorating distressing symptoms, and (c) providing supportive teaching to family and friends. The distresses of forced feeding (nausea, respiratory congestion, diarrhea, edema, etc.) result in discomfort and poor quality of life. The problems of pain, constipation, and depression will definitely reduce intake and if present should already have been addressed. Specific gastrointestinal problems that cause distress and interfere with intake are outlined, along with ways to minimize them, in Table 10.1.

## Relieving Symptoms with Parenteral Hydration

Symptoms such as confusion or mental cloudiness from long-acting metabolites of morphine may be alleviated with hydration. Studies by Bruera and others (Bruera, Franco, Maltoni, Watanabe, & Suarez-Almazor, 1995; Bruera, Macmillan, Kuen, Hanson, & McDonald, 1990) suggest that clysis, or parenteral injection, is preferable over intravenous administration of fluids because it works effectively, is a simpler procedure, and has less potential for infection. A trial of parenteral hydration to relieve confusion is appropriate if it is likely that drug by-product retention is the cause and the patient is not imminently dying. This is particularly important if unfinished business remains.

However, because there are multiple causes of confusion in terminal illness and oral opiates administered in stable regimens are rarely associated with confusion, hydration by IV or clysis should be used only after careful consideration of potential outcomes, degree of value to the patient or family, and duration of benefit. Potential fluid overload and consequent discomfort are highly likely with the multisystem organ failure common at the end of life.

# FAMILY TEACHING

## Understanding Nutritional Needs

The giving of food and fluid has the symbolic importance of love and nurturing. The sharing of food is associated with almost every social event and celebration of our lives. Thus, it is understandably difficult for caregivers and other family members to accept the patient's decreased food and fluid intake during the dying process. It is usually easy for the patient to accept the change due to the discomfort associated with eating. For most caregivers and family members, however, the process involves an adjustment. With education and sensitive communication, acceptance is possible and probable. It is helpful to discuss and have a printed handout presenting the following information:

- Nutritional needs change as illness advances.

# Table 10.1 Interventions to Minimize Gastrointestinal Distress

**TASTE AND SMELL CHANGES**

Avoid foods with offensive odors.

Cold foods such as peanut butter or yogurt may be less objectionable.

Provide good oral hygiene.

The patient may do better if not exposed to odors of food preparation.

**DRY MOUTH**

Saliva substitutes (formulation similar to natural saliva) can be used as needed.

Serve moist foods.

Add gravies or sauces.

Liquids may be sipped as desired.

Frozen juice pops may be appealing.

**SORE THROAT AND MOUTH**

Provide soft, cool foods; avoid temperature extremes.

Avoid acidic, salty, spicy, or hard and crunchy foods.

Assess and treat infections (candidiasis and herpes simplex are common).

Use topical analgesic medications.

**DYSPHAGIA**

Provide the consistency/texture best tolerated.

Feed the portion that best facilitates swallowing (usually small bites).

**NAUSEA AND VOMITING**

Administer indicated medications (e.g., antiemetics, lactase, digestive enzymes).

Avoid foods likely to aggravate nausea, such as fatty, spicy, odorous, or bulky foods.

Avoid physical activity right after eating.

Avoid eating or talking about food in the presence of a patient who is nauseous.

**EARLY SATIETY OR BLOATING**

Offer small, frequent feedings.

Avoid carbonated beverages and gas-producing foods.

**DIARRHEA**

Investigate the role of medications, including bowel stimulants, in causing diarrhea.

Avoid foods known to cause or exacerbate loose stools.

If appropriate, medicate with lactase, pancreatic enzymes, or diphenoxylate/atropine (Lomotil).

◆ Frequently, more than one body system is failing, causing inability of the body to metabolize food normally.

◆ The disease process has altered the patient's desire to eat and ability to digest food, and it has decreased energy levels, changing the experience of eating from a pleasant one to a distressing one.

◆ Food cravings can change from one moment to the next, so a person who provides a requested item should not be personally offended if the patient takes only one or two bites.

◆ Gradual dehydration appears to be a natural way for the body to prevent distressing symptoms such as lung congestion, rattling secretions, shortness of breath, vomiting, edema, and so on.

◆ Because the process of shutting down normal functions is natural, the patient is not "starving"; a dying patient rarely feels hungry or thirsty.

◆ When a patient in advanced stages of disease comes within days of death, it is normal to refuse any intake.

◆ The patient should never be made to feel guilty for "not trying" to eat. Even if the patient wants to eat, he or she often is unable to do so.

## Refocusing Caring Emotions

It is important to stress that caregivers and other family members should not feel powerless because they cannot provide nourishment in the form of food and fluid. They can continue to nourish the patient's mind and spirit with genuine and loving words and gestures, pain control, intellectual stimulation, spiritual guidance, and humor. In this way, the goal of comfort will be achieved.

# THE DILEMMA OF ARTIFICIAL NUTRITION AND HYDRATION IN TERMINAL ILLNESS

Because most hospice patients are followed by their own attending physicians, prescribed therapies can vary widely. They may include intravenous therapies such as chemotherapy, antibiotics, or hydration. Fluids and nourishment provided by a variety of artificial methods are generally perceived by patients, families, and clinicians as being palliative. It is important to understand the fallacy of that belief as it relates to terminally ill patients with multisystem failure. This section provides background information useful in supporting a patient's decision not to have artificial nutrition and hydration (ANH). The information is also helpful for patients in making an informed decision. Patients may have come to believe from past experiences with acute care that to forego ANH will result in discomfort and possibly shorten life expectancy.

## Morality of Caring

Since the time technology has been available to provide ANH, the consensus of the medical and lay communities has been that, even if other medical treatments are foregone in extreme conditions, one must always provide nutrition and hydration. This premise is based on the perceptions that the sustenance of life must always be provided and that dehydration is a distressing state. It is presumed that patients, even those with terminal illnesses, will die sooner without this support. In the past, the legal and moral perception has been that it is not only cruel to "starve someone" but that it is an unusually painful process, equivalent to murder. Providing nourishment has always been a symbol of love and caring and is equated with life itself. Not providing nourishment has been presumed to be inhumane and uncaring. When a patient is dying, the moral obligation felt by any clinician or family member can be very strong. When the certainty of death exists, there is almost always a feeling of failure and the urgent need to provide some intervention to avoid the feeling that one is abandoning the patient. We have come to realize that these presumptions do not hold true in end-stage disease and that there are more realistic ways to show caring.

## Medical Imperatives

Physicians and nurses have been taught that dehydration is a state causing great discomfort and with potential for serious or life-threatening implications. Major medical texts do not discuss dehydration per se; rather, chapters focus on the complexities of body fluids or fluids and electrolytes. Discussions usually begin with an extensive examination of sodium and water metabolism, then go on to consider the metabolism of another important electrolyte, potassium. The implications regarding involvement and breakdown of other physiological functions and systems are complex. Sodium, the major extracellular solute, is particularly important because the sodium and water balance is what controls fluid balance—and ultimately osmolality, electrolyte balance, and acid-base balance.

It has become a medical imperative to monitor and correct these abnormal conditions because doing so is beneficial. In patients with potential for recovery, it may reverse a fatal course. However, in recent years, through hospice experience and research we have come to realize that the pathophysiology of the dying patient may be totally different from that of the patient with potential for recovery. There is evidence that providing ANH may, in fact, cause more discomfort and distressing symptoms than benefit.

## Ethical and Legal Concerns

In 1983, the report of the President's Commission for the Study of Ethical Problems in Medicine and Biomedical and Behavioral Research was published, with many references to a patient's right to refuse treatment. The commission stated that no specific treatments, including usual hospital therapies such as parenteral nutrition or hydration, antibiotics, and transfusions were "universally warranted and thus obligatory for a patient to accept" (p. 90). This was also the year that hospice nurse Joyce Zerwekh's (1983) seminal article "The Dehydration Question" was published, questioning the benefits of artificial hydration in terminal patients.

During the 1980s, numerous court cases and published papers brought attention to the dilemma, with mounting evidence that perhaps more harm than good was resulting from artificial nutrition and hydration in this patient population. In 1986, the American Medical Association published their stance, including nutrition and hydration along with other invasive medical treatments that patients have the right to refuse. The American Dietetic Association and the American Nurses Association followed suit in 1987 and 1988, respectively.

The landmark case *Cruzan v. Director, Missouri Department of Health* (1990) brought a Supreme Court decision on the matter. Justice Sandra Day O'Connor wrote, "Requiring a competent adult to endure such procedures against her will burdens the patient's liberty, dignity, and freedom to determine the course of her own treatment. Accordingly, the liberty guaranteed by the Due Process clause must protect, if it protects anything, an individual's deeply personal decision to reject medical treatments including the artificial delivery of food and water." The challenge, then, is to examine and continually reexamine the issue of what the patient wants and what makes the patient most comfortable. As with any other intervention, the benefits versus the burdens of artificial nutrition and hydration should be explored.

# NUTRITION AND HYDRATION BENEFITS AND BURDENS

## Relationship to Comfort

A number of studies have reported nurses' observations that hospice patients who become dehydrated naturally remain comfortable. In one study (Andrews & Levine, 1989), 80% of hospice nurses surveyed agreed that dehydration is not painful. In the same study, a large majority of the nurses who had witnessed terminal dehydration agreed that dehydration reduces the incidence of distressing symptoms such as vomiting and choking.

In another study (Miller & Albright, 1989), 95% of the hospice nurses believed, from their observations, that aggressive nutritional support is more harmful than beneficial to the patient. The general consensus is that food and fluid should be offered continually but not forced when patients refuse—patients know their own comfort levels.

Some possible explanations for why terminal patients can be comfortable while dehydrated are as follows:

◆ Most of these patients have normal electrolytes despite their dehydration. This type of dehydration is theorized by Billings (1985) to be "eunatremic" rather than hyper- or hyponatremic.

◆ Other variables such as osmolality, BUN (blood urea nitrogen), and creatinine are largely found to be in normal ranges.

◆ Gradual development of dehydration and cachexia simultaneously may be an adaptive process by the body to decrease suffering from imminent death.

◆ Decreased nutritional intake stimulates an increased production of endorphins, a natural analgesic.

◆ Dehydration results in the body's production of dynorphin, also a natural analgesic.

◆ There is rarely a sudden and precipitous drop in intake; in the majority of patients the decrease is gradual, with some intake until the last 2 to 3 days.

## Relationship to Distressing Complications

Many patients who have progressive end-stage disease with multisystem failure and who receive ANH are observed to develop distressing and serious side effects. Numerous studies and reports have documented how hydrating fluids, for nourishment or otherwise, are not physiologically useful. Rather, these fluids produce highly distressing symptoms because the physiologic and metabolic processes of the body are no longer efficient. These symptoms many be summarized as follows:

◆ Fluid overload inhibits release of antidiuretic hormone, which results in increased urinary output, possibly incontinence, or catheterization.

- Increased extracellular fluid (ECF) causes peripheral edema, which results in decreased mobility, increased skin breakdown, and distressing pressure.

- Increased ECF causes pulmonary edema and congestive heart failure, which results in an increase of respiratory secretions, coughing, and dyspnea.

- Increased ECF causes increased gastrointestinal secretions, ascities, pain, nausea, and vomiting.

- Cerebral edema may result in mental disturbance, convulsions, coma, twitching, or hyperirritability.

Well-known changes in physiologic parameters of end-stage cancer, which also may be applicable to other end-stage syndromes, offer some explanation of the lack of beneficial results in this population. Cancer cells replace healthy cells. These cancer cells lose the growth regulatory mechanism and produce massive growths that suppress normal organ function. In addition, these abnormal cells have exponential genetic instability; they divide very rapidly rather than proceeding toward mature differentiation. Therefore, they cannot carry on normal cell function, although there are large numbers of them. Other end-stage syndromes include multiple paraneoplastic syndromes and anaerobic glycolysis, which result in energy deficit and body wasting. Not surprisingly, all of this results in organ malfunction and abnormal responses to interventions.

In addition to metabolic reasons that fluids cause uncomfortable complications, mechanical and physical complications can occur:

- Malnourished patients with terminal illness receiving IV therapy are at risk for sepsis, infiltration, and phlebitis.

- Aspiration pneumonia commonly occurs in terminally ill patients fed with gastric tubes.

- Stomal leakage around enterostomy feeding tubes can result in local infection and/or wound dehiscence (parting of a sutured incision).

- The cost, management, discomfort, and inconvenience of IV therapy in a terminally ill patient could outweigh any potential benefit.

- Diarrhea is a side effect of some tube-feeding formulas.

- General risks of tube feedings include irritation or erosion of nasal passages, esophagus, or stomach.

- If restraints are needed to prevent the patient from pulling out tubes or IV lines, this sets up another cascade of problems.

## Relationship to Longevity

Finally, there is no evidence that IV therapy of this sort in patients who are terminally ill serves to prolong life. However, even if there were, it would be inappropriate and unethical to study the issue by dividing patients with end-stage disease into two groups, giving one group ANH and withholding it from the second group. However, several retrospective studies (summarized in Smith, 1997) show that patients without IV support live as long or longer than those who have IV support. One can conclude from this evidence that the patient will die from the disease process regardless of degree of intake.

### REFERENCES AND SUGGESTED READINGS

American Dietetic Association. (1987). Position of the American Dietetic Association: Issues in feeding the terminally ill adult. *Journal of the American Dietetic Association, 87*(1), 78–85.

American Medical Association. (1986). *Withholding or withdrawing life prolonging medical treatment.* Chicago: Author.

American Nurses Association. (1988). Withdrawing or withholding food and fluid: Guidelines of the ANA Committee on Ethics. *American Journal of Nursing, 88,* 797–798.

American Nurses Association. (1992). *Foregoing artificial nutrition and hydration* (Position Statement). Washington, DC: Author.

Andrews, M. R., Bell, E. R., Smith, S. A., Tischler, J., & Veglia, J. M. (1993). Dehydration in terminally ill patients: Is it appropriate palliative care? *Postgraduate Medicine, 93*(1), 201–206.

Andrews, M. R., & Levine, A. M. (1989). Dehydration in the terminal patient: Perception of hospice nurses. *American Journal of Hospice Care, 6*(1), 31–34.

Billings, A. (1985). Comfort measures for the terminally ill: Is dehydration painful? *Journal of the American Geriatric Society, 33*(11), 808–810.

Boyle, D. M., Abernathy, G., Baker, L., & Wall, A. C. (1988). End-of-life confusion in patients with cancer. *Oncology Nursing Forum, 25,* 1335–1343.

Bruera, E., Franco, J. J., Maltoni, M., Watanabe, S., & Suarez-Almazor, M. (1995). Changing pattern of agitated impaired mental status in patients with advanced cancer: Association with cognitive monitoring, hydration, and opioid rotation. *Journal of Pain and Symptom Management, 10*(4), 287–291.

Bruera, E., Macmillan, K., Kuen, N., Hanson, J., & McDonald, R. N. (1990). A controlled trial of megesterol acetate on appetite, caloric intake, nutritional status, and other symptoms in patients with advanced cancer. *Cancer, 66,* 1279–1282.

Burge, F. I. (1993). Dehydration symptoms of palliative care cancer patients. *Journal of Pain and Symptom Management, 8*(7), 454–464.

Burge, F. I., King, D. B., & Willison, D. (1990). Intravenous fluids and the hospitalized dying: A medical last rite? *Canadian Family Physician, 36,* 883–886.

Cruzan v. Director, Missouri Department of Health, 110 S. Ct. 2841 (1990).

Gallagher-Allred, C. R. (1991). Nutritional care of the terminally ill patient and family. In J. Penson & R. Fisher (Eds.), *Palliative care for people with cancer.* London: Hodder and Stoughton.

Gallagher-Allred, C. R. (1989). *Nutritional care of the terminally ill.* Rockville, MD: Aspen.

Gallagher-Allred, C. R., & Amenta, M. O. (Eds.). (1993). *Nutrition and hydration in hospice care*. New York: Haworth Press.

House, N. (1992, October). The hydration question: Hydration or dehydration of terminally ill patients. *Professional Nurse*, pp. 44–48.

Lynn, J., & Harrold, J. (1999). *Handbook for mortals: Guidance for people facing serious illness*. New York: Oxford University Press.

McCann, R. M., Hall, W. J., & Groth-Juncker, A. (1994). Comfort care for terminally ill patients: The appropriate use of nutrition and hydration. *Journal of the American Medical Association, 272*, 1263–1266.

Meares, C. J. (1994). Terminal dehydration: A review. *American Journal of Hospice and Palliative Care, 11*(3), 10–14.

Miller, R. J., & Albright, P. G. (1989). What is the role of nutritional support and hydration in terminal cancer patients? *American Journal of Hospice Care, 6*(6), 33–38.

Musgrave, C. F. (1990). Terminal dehydration: To give or not to give intravenous fluid? *Cancer Nursing, 13*(1), 62–66.

National Conference of Catholic Bishops' Committee. (1992, April 2). Nutrition and hydration: Moral and pastoral reflections. *Catholic News*, p. 18.

President's Commission for the Study of Ethical Problems in Medicine and Biomedical and Behavioral Research. (1983). *Deciding to forego life-sustaining treatment*. Washington, DC: U.S. Government Printing Office.

Printz, L. A. (1988). Is withholding hydration a valid comfort measure in the terminally ill? *Geriatrics, 43*(11), 84–88.

Printz, L. A. (1992). Terminal dehydration: A compassionate treatment. *Archives of Internal Medicine, 152*, 697–700.

Rousseau, P. C. (1991). How fluid deprivation affects the terminally ill. *RN, 55*(1), 73–76.

Smith, S. (1995). Patient-induced dehydration: Can it ever be therapeutic? *Oncology Nursing Forum, 22*, 1487–1491.

Smith, S. (1997). Controversies in hydrating the terminally ill patient. *Journal of Intravenous Nursing, 20*(4), 193–200.

Vullo-Navich, K., Smith, S., Andrews, M., Levine, A. M., Tischler, J. F., & Veglia, J. M. (1998). Comfort and incidence of abnormal serum sodium, BUN, creatinine, and osmolality in dehydration of terminal illness. *American Journal of Hospice and Palliative Care, 15*(2), 77–84.

Waller, A., Hershkowitz, M., & Adunsky, A. (1994). The effect of intravenous fluid infusion on blood and urine parameters of hydration and on state of consciousness in terminal cancer patients. *American Journal of Hospice and Palliative Care, 61*(4), 26–29.

Zerwekh, J. V. (1983). The dehydration question. *Nursing 83, 13*(1), 47–51.

Zerwekh, J.V. (1997). Do dying patients really need IV fluids? *American Journal of Nursing, 97*(3), 26–30.

# CHAPTER 11

# Legal and Ethical Issues

**PURPOSE**

The purpose of this chapter is to describe the major legal mandates and ethical dilemmas relative to hospice care. Specific documents and ethical approaches will be discussed.

**OBJECTIVES**

Upon completion of this chapter, the learner will be able to:

1. Discuss the ethical dilemmas in health care that led to palliative care reform

2. Discuss legislation related to informed consent and refusal of treatment

3. Define the ethical principles applicable to health care

**CONTENT OUTLINE**

I. Legal Processes Affecting Terminal Care

    A. Movement toward palliative care reform

    B. President's Commission

    C. Supreme Court decision

    D. Self-Determination Act

II. Documenting Patient Wishes

    A. Informed consent

    B. Durable power of attorney for health care/health care proxy

    C. Living will

    D. Do not resuscitate (DNR)

    E. Treatment instructions

III. Other Laws Related to Hospice

    A.  Death pronouncement and nurse practice acts

    B.  Controlled substances

    C.  Hospice licensure and certification

IV. Ethical Issues

    A.  Ethical principles applicable to health care

    B.  Ethical issues in hospice care

# LEGAL PROCESSES AFFECTING TERMINAL CARE

## Movement toward Palliative Care Reform

Supreme Court Justice Sandra Day O'Conner, in giving her concurring opinion in *Cruzan v. Director, Missouri Department of Health* (1990), stated that a seriously ill or dying patient whose wishes are not honored may feel a captive of the machinery required for life-sustaining measures or other medical interventions. The majority opinion in that case was that any competent adult may refuse any treatment, including life-sustaining treatment. Why would such a case come before the Supreme Court? Shouldn't health care providers make those kinds of decisions?

As technology and medical treatments mushroomed in our country, it was expected that any available intervention should be tried. As intervention became a standard of practice, futile treatment in progressive incurable illness became commonplace. During this same time, less attention was given to informed consent, patient values, and pain management. Many people came to fear overtreatment of disease, with no benefit and great discomfort, and undertreatment of physical and emotional pain. As individual rights have become a popular societal theme, self-determination rights have extended to health care as well. The following discussion highlights some of the major activities impacting this change.

## President's Commission

When the report of the President's Commission for the Study of Ethical Problems in Medicine and Biomedical and Behavioral Research was published in 1983, it brought to public attention the inherent right of every patient to be informed about and involved in health care decisions. The report specifically discussed the issue of cardiopulmonary resuscitation (CPR) as a very painful and intrusive procedure and stated that all patients have the right to decide if CPR, or other life-sustaining treatments, should be part of their plan of care.

## Supreme Court Decision

In June of 1990, the Supreme Court handed down the Cruzan decision, affirming a competent adult's right to refuse medical treatment. The ruling upholds the constitutional right to liberty as implying the right to reject unwanted treatment, whether one is terminally ill or not. It states that competent persons generally are permitted to refuse medical treatment, even at the risk of death. The ruling also specifies that medical treatment includes the artificial delivery of food and water.

## Self-Determination Act

Later in 1990, Congress passed a public law, effective December 1991, requiring all health care providers reimbursed by Medicare or Medicaid to provide all patients with information about their rights to be involved in decision making and to develop methods of documenting patients' wishes. Commonly referred to as the Patient Self-Determination Act, this law mandates that health care facilities educate professionals and consumers on the topic of advance directives. Unfortunately, some facilities have misinterpreted this mandate to mean the patient must have an advance directive before entering the system. This was not the intent. The public law requires only that information be provided and that, if the patient does execute an advance directive, it become a part of the medical record and the patient's wishes be honored.

# DOCUMENTING PATIENT WISHES

## Informed Consent

Based on Supreme Court rulings and federal legislation, there is no question that patients have the moral, ethical, and legal right to receive full information about their conditions and treatment options. For patients with a terminal condition, this must include pertinent information—for example, that negative outcomes may result from CPR, that foregoing artificial nutrition and hydration will not necessarily be distressing, and that a course of chemotherapy may not affect survival time significantly.

It is obvious that information should be given with a great deal of sensitivity and compassion, but it is imperative that the information be complete. No patient should ever be asked to begin a therapy or discontinue a therapy without adequate information about potential benefits and burdens. For a patient to make a treatment choice with true informed consent, options and outcomes must be clearly explained. Beyond this, the patient's interest or queries should guide the provision of additional information.

Acknowledging when the focus of care has shifted from treatment to palliation and communicating that to the patient and family are never easy tasks. However, when cure is no longer possible and the patient has a limited time, the patient has certain rights. Table 11.1 lists generally accepted rights of a terminally ill patient from a moral and ethical perspective.

Patients entering hospice are asked to sign a consent for a palliative focus of treatment. Although these documents may vary in wording, most include some statement about shifting the focus from curative, aggressive measures to palliative or comfort care. Whether care will be provided at home or in an inpatient setting, discussions need to address patient and family goals and describe what the particular hospice program can offer. Patients referred to hospice for the first time will need an explanation of the palliative nature of hospice and how it is different from acute care. (Do not presume patients have been given this information.) Should a patient desire an aggressive course of cure-oriented treatment, it should be made clear that hospice is not an appropriate program to fulfill that wish.

Sometimes patients and their families perceive entering a hospice program to be just as traumatic as first learning the diagnosis. There will be a period of adjustment requiring support, patience, and sensitive provision of information in increments the patient and family can handle. Hospice staff must engage in a continuing discussion with the patient and family/significant other about the course of the patient's illness and the quality-of-life measures that are available. Ongoing explanations of disease progression and changing options are essential for the patient and family to make further informed decisions and to cope with the patient's decline.

Next described are a variety of methods by which patients may document their wishes. The terminology may vary slightly with various state laws but, generally, every person has the right to name a surrogate decision maker, to refuse resuscitation and life support, and to leave specific instructions for treatment if one is unable to speak for oneself. Collectively, the documents representing the patient's wishes are known as *advance directives*.

## Durable Power of Attorney for Health Care/Health Care Proxy

Whether it is called *durable power of attorney for health care* or *health care proxy*, every state has some statute or public law for the provision

## Table 11.1   Patient Rights in Terminal Illness

1. RIGHT TO KNOW THE TRUTH
   —*about condition, prognosis, and options*
2. RIGHT TO CONSENT TO OR REFUSE TREATMENT
   —*with input into plan of care*
3. RIGHT TO EXPERT CARE
   —*to alleviate emotional and physical symptoms*
4. RIGHT TO CONFIDENTIALITY AND PRIVACY
   —*and respect for personal values*
5. RIGHT TO CONTROL ENVIRONMENT AND SETTING
   —*for the final days of life*
6. RIGHT TO DETERMINE CARE
   —*and disposition of the body upon death*

of surrogate decision making when a patient becomes unable to do so. The next of kin can be a decision maker without filling out and signing a form, but in some cases the patient may prefer someone other than the next of kin to be the surrogate. That wish can be honored only if the patient has signed a document to that effect while still competent.

Some points to remember about health care proxy are as follows:

♦ The person named as health care proxy supersedes next of kin.

♦ The patient may choose anyone who is 18 years old or older and competent.

♦ In most states these forms do not have to be notarized.

♦ Witnesses on the form cannot be relatives or beneficiaries.

♦ The patient can also include specific directions for care in specific situations.

♦ A general power of attorney is usually for fiscal and personal matters but can include health care decisions if specifically outlined.

♦ Once filled out, signed, and properly witnessed, in most states the directive is valid until revoked by the patient.

## Living Will

The living will is another advance directive in which the patient specifies under what circumstances he or she would no longer want aggressive or life-sustaining interventions. Most living will forms are worded in a general way—for example, "I only want comfort measures if I have a terminal condition without hope of recovery." This leaves a lot open to interpretation, including what constitutes comfort measures. Thus, individuals should be encouraged to have full information on their conditions, prognoses, and options so they can think through specific instructions that are important to them.

When health care providers know a patient has an advance directive, they should read it carefully because each directive will be different; nothing should be presumed. For example, one patient may not want any invasive treatment but may wish to be resuscitated. Another may wish antibiotics but no other IV therapy. Sometimes inconsistencies will appear, indicating the patient is not clear about his or her condition, options, and potential outcomes. Patients may need help in understanding what they have chosen and may want to revise the document.

## Do Not Resuscitate (DNR)

Hospice programs must assure that a patient's right not to be resuscitated is protected. This requires vigilance to assure that a do-not-resuscitate (DNR) request is clearly documented and reordered as often as policy dictates. Communication with inpatient units, transportation systems, and emergency medical services must be clear to prevent unwanted CPR.

To prevent inappropriate use of emergency calls (i.e., 911 calls), patients and families should be prepared for anticipated emergencies, including the patient's death, and rehearse actions to take. Such preparation is essential in states that do not have legislation relating to out-of-hospital DNR status. Hospice staff should also communicate with local emergency rooms and emergency medical technicians, as well as with legislators, to encourage understanding of the challenge and to recommend public policy changes that may be necessary to protect patients' rights.

If the patient wishes hospice care but still requests CPR, the hospice staff should initiate discussions regarding benefits and burdens of CPR to facilitate an informed decision. If the patient or surrogate persists in requesting CPR, staff must communicate that resuscitation and continuing life support are inimical to the hospice mission and will not be performed by the hospice staff. Patients may not, according to National Hospice Organization standards, be refused hospice care in this case, but they do need to be guided in making plans to secure that particular service elsewhere. Very few patients persist in this request as they experience a decline in their conditions.

## Treatment Instructions

Although a DNR order, a living will, and hospice consent all imply no aggressive curative treatments, the patient must be assured that this does not mean "no treatment." The patient needs to know that hospice care is a specialized treatment program actively addressing all the needs of the terminally ill. Further, patients should be encouraged to put into writing specific wishes about care they would or would not want to receive and to describe what "quality of life" means to them. These instructions help caregivers and surrogate decision makers know best how to honor the patient's wishes. This type of advance directive is very important if the patient receives terminal care in a nonhospice setting. It should also be noted that there are many forms available that incorporate such care instructions along with all of the advance directives previously discussed.

# OTHER LAWS RELATED TO HOSPICE

## Death Pronouncement and Nurse Practice Acts

Most states now have legislation permitting death pronouncement by registered nurses. Laws vary from state to state as to specific nomenclature and specific guidelines. For example, in Pennsylvania a registered nurse may assess death but cannot determine the cause of death. In Pennsylvania the law also specifies that the registered nurse assessing death must be one who is involved in direct care of the patient and that the death must have been anticipated. In other states, the registered nurse cannot pronounce the patient dead but can report to the physician the absence of vital signs. Practices will also vary from county to county within the same state as to who contacts whom and in what order. It is imperative that nurses be responsible for knowing and adhering to these and other provisions of the law as defined in the nurse practice acts of their state.

## Controlled Substances

Because the problem of abuse or illicit use of narcotics is so great, laws governing their ordering, dispensing, and disposal are detailed and very strict. Only physicians can order controlled substances, and only pharmacists or physicians can dispense them. A new order must be written before any change in the dose. Every health care organization has the responsibility to develop written policies regarding disposal of any controlled substance not used by the patient.

Although there are good reasons for strict laws to control drugs with high abuse potential, currently the opposite concern also exists: that regulatory policies such as triplicate prescription programs and limitation on number of doses are discouraging physician prescribing, resulting in inadequate pain management.

## Hospice Licensure and Certification

All hospice programs wishing to be reimbursed by Medicare must go through a program and be designated "Medicare approved." Many states now have a certification process in place. Some will accept Medicare certification as qualifying for state certification. Other states have even more stringent requirements than does Medicare.

# ETHICAL ISSUES

## Ethical Principles Applicable to Health Care

Ethics is the study of moral issues. We speak of moral or ethical dilemmas because these are situations that have no right or wrong answers. These issues usually affect individuals on a deeply personal level, and most people have very strong opinions resulting from their own unique values. When these dilemmas arise, we are obliged to apply all pertinent laws and ethical principles in weighing the pros and cons of potential decisions.

The main ethical principles applicable to health care may be defined briefly as follows:

- ◆ Autonomy: Respecting the rights of the patient or surrogates to refuse or accept treatment options and the scope of care

- ◆ Truth telling (veracity): Openness and honesty in providing the patient with information necessary to give informed consent or in providing further information requested by the patient

- ◆ Confidentiality: Respect for the privacy of each patient, with personal or medical information shared only among team members for the sole purpose of appropriate care planning

- ◆ Nonmaleficence: "Do no harm"—the avoidance of harm or injury to the patient

- ◆ Beneficence: Acting for the good of, or in the best interest of, the patient

- ◆ Distributive justice: Equality of access to and distribution of health care resources

+ Professional integrity: The right and responsibility of health care practitioners to establish and uphold quality standards of practice and not to act contrary to such

## Ethical Issues in Hospice Care

Increasingly, issues have been recognized as being derivatives of terminal illness care and associated concerns of society. Every hospice program has a responsibility to acknowledge and establish parameters covering the ethical issues inherent in the care of the dying. In addition to the topics discussed in this chapter, ethical issues concern such matters as futile treatments at the end of life, distributive justice, and euthanasia/physician-assisted suicide.

Futile treatments at the end of life have become commonplace in our society. In part, the situation arises from the availability of pharmaceuticals, procedures, and high-tech equipment—in part, from a medical and public ethic that values life and honors the code of doing everything possible. Unfortunately, for patients who are no longer responding to the usual treatments, these efforts result in more burdens than benefits. What is needed is a new perspective that would view patients' goals and values at this point in life, then consider how the knowledge of medical science can be applied to meet those goals. Respecting patient autonomy, practicing beneficence, and truth telling would all come together to enhance comfort and quality of life.

Distributive justice would ensure that all citizens would have equal access to appropriate health care resources. For patients who have incurable, life-threatening illnesses, justice means access to quality, comprehensive end-of-life palliative care. Deterrents to this goal include lack of insurance coverage, inadequate guidelines by managed care organizations, and lack of knowledge among professionals about palliative care. A major obstacle is the high value we place on technology in health care in the United States. This high-tech care gets reimbursed, futile or not, while cost containment efforts cut low profile services such as home care and psychological support.

Euthanasia and physician-assisted suicide are not condoned in hospice and palliative care. There may be those who perceive lack of aggressive curative therapies as a form of euthanasia. What needs to be made clear is that, although palliative care does focus on methods to make an expected death less painful, no action intended to hasten death is acceptable. Nonmaleficence means avoiding harm to the patient. This includes avoiding actions that add to suffering or that would directly cause death. Physician-assisted suicide is illegal in the United States, except in the state of Oregon, and even there the law continues to be contested. It is the hope of hospice and palliative care providers that by alleviating pain and other physical and mental distresses, patients will not feel so desperate as to seek suicide.

Thus we can see that the challenge to improve end-of-life care in this country is not to seek new miracles, but rather to learn to use existing therapies in a new way. We need to work at improving end-of-life education in nursing and medical schools, break down the legal and bureaucratic obstacles to equal access to care, and redefine goals so that palliative care for incurable illness is valued and reimbursed.

## REFERENCES AND SUGGESTED READINGS

Bresica, F. J. (1993). Specialized care of the terminally ill. In V. T. Devita, S. Hellman, & S. A. Rosenberg (Eds.), *Cancer: Principles and practice of oncology* (4th ed.). Philadelphia: J. B. Lippincott.

Buccheri, G. F., Ferrigno, D., Curcio, A., Vola, F., & Rossa, A. (1989). Continuation of chemotherapy versus supportive care alone in patients with inoperable non–small cell lung cancer and stable disease after two or three cycles of MACC: Results of a randomized prospective trial. *Cancer, 63*,428–432.

Burge, F. L., King, D. B., & Willison, D. (1990). Intravenous fluids and the hospitalized dying: A medical last rite? *Canadian Family Physician, 36,* 883–886.

Byock, I. R. (1992). Cancer chemotherapy and the boundaries of the hospice model. *American Journal of Hospice and Palliative Care, 9*(2), 4–5.

Byock, I. R. (1994). Ethics from a hospice perspective. *American Journal of Hospice and Palliative Care, 11*(4), 9–11.

Callahan, D. (1991). Rationing medical progress: The way to affordable health care. *New England Journal of Medicine, 322,* 1810–1813.

Callahan, D. (1993). *The troubled dream of life: In search of a peaceful death.* New York: Simon and Schuster.

Cellerino, R., Tummarello, D., Guidi, F., Isidori, P., Raspugii, M., Biscottini, B., & Fatati, G. (1991). A randomized trial of alternating chemotherapy versus best supportive care in advanced non–small cell lung cancer. *Journal of Clinical Oncology, 9,* 1453–1461.

Cruzan v. Director, Missouri Department of Health. 110 S. Ct. 2841 (1990).

Cundiff, D. (1992). *Euthanasia is not the answer: A hospice physician's view.* Totowa, NJ: Humana Press.

Faber-Langendoen, K. (1991). Resuscitation of patients with metastatic cancer: Is transient benefit still futile? *Archives of Internal Medicine, 151,* 235–239.

Field, M. J., & Cassel, C. K. (Eds.). (1997). *Approaching death: Improving care at the end of life.* Washington, DC: National Academy Press.

The Hastings Center. (1987). *Guidelines on the termination of life sustaining treatment and the care of the dying.* Indianapolis: Indiana University Press.

*Hospice ethics: An education resource paper.* (1995). Office of Geriatrics and Extended Care, Office of Academic Affairs, Veteran's Administration Central Office, Washington, DC.

Lamerton, R. (1991). Dehydration in dying patients. *Lancet, 337,* 981–982.

Lynn, J., & Harrold, J. (1999). *Handbook for mortals: Guidance for people facing serious illness.* New York: Oxford University Press.

Lynn, T. (1985). Ethics in hospice care. In *Hospice handbook: A guide for managers and planners*. Rockville, MD: Aspen.

Miller, R. J. (1989). The role of chemotherapy in the hospice patient. *American Journal of Hospice Care, 6*(3), 19–26.

National Hospice Organization. (1993). *Discontinuation of hospice care: Ethical issues*. South Deerfield, MA: Author.

Patient Self-Determination Act, § 4206 & 4751, Omnibus Budget Reconciliation Act of 1990, Public Law 101–508 (1991).

President's Commission for the Study of Ethical Problems in Medicine and Biomedical and Behavioral Research. (1983). *Deciding to forego life-sustaining treatment*. Washington, DC: U.S. Government Printing Office.

Smith, S. A. (1997). Controversies in hydrating the terminally ill patient. *Journal of Intravenous Nursing, 20*(4), 193–200.

# CHAPTER 12

# Continuity of Care and the Medicare Hospice Benefit

**PURPOSE**

The purpose of this chapter is to describe the multiple liaisons necessary for continuity of care and discuss how Medicare defines hospice services.

**OBJECTIVES**

Upon completion of this chapter, the learner will be able to:

1. Discuss the liaisons necessary for continuity of care

2. Explain why Medicare plays a major role in determining hospice practices

3. List some of the major program requirements of a Medicare-approved hospice program

**CONTENT OUTLINE**

I. Liaisons Necessary for Continuity of Care

    A.  Other hospices

    B.  Community agencies

    C.  Physicians

    D.  Inpatient settings

II. Overview of the Medicare Hospice Benefit

    A.  Background

B.  Program requirements

C.  Patient eligibility

D.  Levels of care

E.  Benefit periods

F.  Challenges for the future

# LIAISONS NECESSARY FOR CONTINUITY OF CARE

Because the goals and philosophy of hospice care are distinctly different than those of acute care, it is important that the same quality of specialized hospice care be provided regardless of setting or clinicians involved. This continuity, or consistency, takes conscious effort on the part of the primary provider of hospice services. The crux of the matter is to ensure that patient wishes and the plan of care agreed upon are known and honored from the beginning of care to the end. To make this happen, liaisons with other hospices, community agencies, physicians, and inpatient settings must be developed.

### Other hospices

Because the majority of hospice programs are now Medicare approved, certain policies and services are assumed to be similar. Even so, if patients transfer from one hospice to another, effective communication is necessary to convey patient/family values and goals of care. Some commonly seen variations among hospices relate to policies on resuscitation, inpatient care, volunteer services, and bereavement services. If a Veterans Administration (VA) medical center hospice program is involved, it is important to know that federal policy does not allow VAs to collect Medicare, and therefore VA hospice programs cannot be Medicare certified. It is also of interest that although all VAs are mandated to make hospice care an option for terminally ill patients, there is no consistency in how each medical center carries this out. Some will have inpatient units, and others will not. A few VAs supervise their own home care, but most will refer their patients to hospice programs in the community for home care.

### Community agencies

Liaison with other agencies that provide services and/or instructions to patients are important to ensure consistency in goals and philosophy. Such agencies might include medical equipment providers, therapists, or social service agencies.

*Physicians*

The dictionary defines *liaison* as a contact maintained by communication in order to assure concerted action and cooperation. Each contact with a physician is an opportunity to convey the goals and philosophy of the patient, as well as insight into the hospice perception of palliation. Hospice team members must be patiently persistent in this effort, remembering that most physicians have little exposure to hospice and a great deal of daily exposure to acute, aggressive philosophies.

*Inpatient settings*

If a hospice program does not have its own inpatient unit, beds for inpatient care are contracted for with a hospital, nursing home, or another hospice's inpatient unit. The important details unique to hospice care will be included in a written contract. The sharing of policies, procedures, and reference materials can strengthen the liaison. Offers to provide inservices or other educational programs will enhance continuity.

## OVERVIEW OF THE MEDICARE HOSPICE BENEFIT

### Background

In the early years of hospice growth in America, it became obvious that reliable, consistent funding would be necessary for program survival. Concerted campaigning for federal reimbursement was successful in August of 1982, when legislation was passed to include hospice care as an option for terminal illness in Medicare beneficiaries. The Medicare Hospice Benefit went into effect in 1983 on a trial basis and was made permanent in 1986. The benefit is an option for Medicare Part A beneficiaries who have a terminal diagnosis and a prognosis of 6 months or less.

As with all Medicare benefits, the Medicare Hospice Benefit is administered by the Health Care Financing Administration (HCFA), a division of the Department of Health and Human Services. Any changes in policy come about only when Congress approves new legislation. Another level for administration of the Medicare Hospice Benefit is that of fiscal intermediaries. Intermediaries are usually regional or national health care managers or insurance companies who vie for the job of handling the billing for Medicare in the various regions of the country. Hospices wishing to be Medicare approved are surveyed to evaluate compliance with pertinent regulations, monitored on an ongoing basis, and periodically reevaluated. There are additional reviews and audits if specific problems are identified.

Because Medicare is the primary funding source for hospice programs, Medicare requirements have become the standard for hospice care in America. Fortunately, HCFA has been responsive to concerted efforts of the National Hospice Organization and other interest groups to maintain an ongoing dialogue between those who make the laws and those who carry them out in the clinical setting. Most non-federal third-party health care insurers and state Medicaid programs generally adopt policies in line with Medicare.

## Program Requirements

There are certain services all hospice programs must provide if they are Medicare approved. Although the dollar amount of reimbursement varies depending on the level of care the patient is receiving and the location the service is delivered, the program is expected to provide all services without extra billing for any particular service. Table 12.1 summarizes the basic services; these are applicable only to the terminal illness, not to other diagnoses the patient may have.

In addition to what the patient can expect, numerous other regulations define agency practices with regard to billing, documentation, and reporting. Some of the program regulations are as follows:

+ A total of 80% of care days must be home care (this figure reflects cumulative care days for all patients, not days for each individual patient).

+ The physician must document certification of terminal diagnosis and limited prognosis at the beginning of each benefit period.

+ Certain services are designated "core services," meaning they must be provided by the agency, not contracted. Core services are nursing, social services, and counseling. Prior to August 5, 1997, physician services were also on the list, but these now may be contracted.

+ A Medicare-approved hospice program must provide the same services to every patient, regardless of payment source.

+ Provisions must be made for continuity of care, informed consent, and quality assurance monitoring.

+ Each agency is responsible for having a written policy on handling and disposing of narcotics.

+ Volunteers are a program requirement and must provide 5% of all patient hours.

## Table 12.1   Mandated Medicare Hospice Services

Nursing care

Medical supplies, appliances, and durable medical equipment (DME)

Prescribed medications

Physician services

Home health aides and homemaker services

Physical, occupational, and other therapies as indicated

Medical social services

Dietary and other counseling

Inpatient care

Respite care (up to 5 days)

Interdisciplinary team care

Bereavement support for at least 12 months

Palliative treatments ordered by attending physicians

Around-the-clock availability for emergencies

Diagnostic studies indicated for comfort care

## Patient Eligibility

Medicare coverage for hospice care is available if (a) the patient is eligible for Medicare Part A; (b) the patient's doctor and the hospice medical director certify that the patient is terminally ill, with a life expectancy of 6 months or less if the disease runs its normal course; (c) the patient signs a statement (election) choosing hospice care instead of standard Medicare benefits for the terminal illness; and (d) the care is provided by a Medicare-approved hospice program. The coverage is under Medicare Part A, usually reserved for inpatient hospital care, because it is perceived as a replacement for inpatient care. (The patient's attending physician continues to bill Medicare Part B for professional services.) As of 1993, patients who opted for the benefit represented the following categories of disease: cancer 78%, cardiac 10%, AIDS 4%, renal 1%, Alzheimer's 1%, and miscellaneous others 6% (Berry, Zeri, & Egan, 1997).

To make an informed decision, patients should be made aware of some further facts. Patients need to understand that the focus in hospice is on care, comfort, and quality of life, not on curing the disease. As opposed to standard Medicare home health services, patients do not have to be home-bound to qualify for home care; they are, in fact, encouraged to participate in all activities as they are able. It is very important for patients to understand that hospice services apply only to care of symptoms related to the terminal diagnosis, not to other conditions. Patients need to know they have the option of continuing to be followed by their current physicians. Many patients wonder if their Social Security or other retirement payments are affected when they enter a Medicare hospice program; they need to know these benefits will not change.

Patients have the right to cancel (revoke) the hospice benefit at any time and return to standard Medicare coverage for the terminal condition. If patients later decide to reenter the hospice program, they may do so and begin a new period of coverage if they meet the certification requirement.

## Levels of Care

*Routine home care* is most frequently the level of care indicated. It includes all home visits and needed supplies, medications, and other indicated services. Routine home care involves the family or significant others, as well as volunteers and professionals from various disciplines.

*Continuous home care* is usually related to a period of medical crisis, requiring more extensive care to manage acute symptoms. This level of care is defined as provision of continuous care at least 8 hours of the day by licensed nurses. It is the hope that this level of care can prevent unnecessary inpatient stays.

*Inpatient care* is required when acute pain or other symptoms cannot be managed in the home setting. It is usually a short-term admission, with the average length of stay being 5 to 7 days. The hospice program may have its own inpatient unit, or it may contract beds with a hospital, long-term care facility, or skilled nursing facility. The hospice program is responsible for the cost of the inpatient stay.

*Inpatient respite care* is the level of care designed to provide a brief respite (usually 5 days) for the primary caregiver. The admission is usually at the same site a hospice program would use for general inpatient care, but this admission does not need to meet the same criteria. Many primary caregivers have the sole responsibility for the patient around the clock and are likely overextended and lacking adequate rest. The respite permits rest and emotional rejuvenation.

## Benefit Periods

As Congress passes legislation proposed by HCFA for changes in the Medicare Hospice Benefit, the benefit periods will vary. As of August 1997, the benefit periods are two 90-day periods followed by an indefinite number of 60-day periods. Previously, if patients dropped the hospice benefit, not only did they lose the remaining days in that period, if they were in the last period when they revoked the benefit, they lost all opportunity of returning to the hospice program. The advantage of the newer benefit arrangement is that patients can always come back to a new 60-day period if they meet the eligibility requirements.

The benefit periods may be used consecutively or at intervals. Regardless of whether the periods are used one right after the other or at different times, the patient must be certified as terminally ill, with an expected prognosis of 6 months or less, at the beginning of each period.

## Challenges for the Future

Can specialized hospice care survive without compromising its founding tenets and high ideals of quality and cost-saving care at the end of life? There are challenges to be faced:

- Requirements imposed by third-party payers without adequate reimbursement to carry them out and other financial inequities that threaten survival of programs

- Differences in the definition of *palliation* between hospice as a specialty and palliative care as a specialty

- Disparity between hospice philosophy and the philosophy of the nonhospice physicians who follow hospice patients

- Late referrals, which rob patients and families of the opportunity to benefit from the program

- Lack of access to hospice for end-of-life care for many segments of the population (e.g., minorities, the uninsured)

- Disagreement among physicians, Medicare, and other third-party insurers as to the most appropriate method of determining prognosis (especially with the noncancer diagnoses)

A number of activities are being pursued by hospices to address these challenges. Hospices are realizing that their chief executive officers need to be expert fiscal managers to remain in competition with other health care providers, as well as being astute at developing beneficial networks and alliances. This means adopting business practices with the potential for reducing costs while improving productivity and quality of care.

One of the ways in which hospice programs have cut costs is by forming alliances, and as groups, working on cost-cutting approaches. These approaches may include development of effective but low-cost protocols, negotiations for volume discounts, or operation of their own hospice pharmacies. Independent businesses are springing up to become group providers for hospice programs. Some alliances are working not only on improving cost effectiveness of hospice care, but also on improving visibility, quality of care, public education, and hospice advocacy.

Education and promotional activities include renewed interest in research, curriculum development for various disciplines, involvement in public policy, and interactive learning processes with other health care arenas. Proactive initiatives through local, state, and national organizations can enhance public opinion of hospice as a unique specialized care option for patients diagnosed with a terminal illness.

### REFERENCES AND SUGGESTED READINGS

Berry, P., Zeri, K., & Egan, K. (1997). *The hospice nurse's study guide: A preparation for the CRNH candidate.* Pittsburgh: Hospice and Palliative Nurses Association.

Mahoney, J. J. (1996). Inclusion in American healthcare. In D. C. Sheehan & W. B. Forman, *Hospice and palliative care: Concepts and practice.* Boston: Jones and Bartlett.

National Hospice Organization. (1998). *Hospice care: A physician's guide.* Arlington, VA: Author.

National Hospice Organization. (1993, October). National hospice profile. *Newsline,* p. 2.

National Hospice Organization. (1993). *Standards of a hospice program of care.* Arlington, VA: Author.

U.S. Department of Health and Human Services. (1997). *Interpretive guidelines: Hospices.* Washington, DC: Author.

U.S. Department of Health and Human Services, Department of Commerce National Technical Information Services. (1997). *Medicare: Hospice manual.* Washington, DC: Author.

Veterans Health Administration, Department of Veterans Affairs. (1992). *Directive 10–92–091: Policy on implementation of hospice programs.* Washington, DC: Author.

# APPENDIX A

# Chapter Tests

# Hospice Philosophy, History, and Goals

1. Concerning the historical development of hospice, select the one correct statement from the following list:

   a. the first hospice in the United States was St. Christopher's in Philadelphia

   b. hospice is a new concept, begun in the 1970s

   c. the Connecticut Hospice was founded in 1974

   d. we now have 868 hospice programs in the United States

2. Which one of the following statements appropriately describes the philosophy of hospice care?

   a. hospice philosophy hastens the patient's death, especially through the use of pain medications

   b. hospice philosophy helps the patient to give up hope

   c. hospice philosophy delays the patient's death so he or she can get affairs in order

   d. hospice philosophy considers the patient and family the unit of care

3. The founder of the modern hospice movement was:

   a. Dr. Avery Wiseman

   b. Dr. Cicely Saunders

   c. Dr. Elisabeth Kübler-Ross

   d. Dr. Herman Feifel

4. The field of thanatology is the study of:

   a. religious orders

   b. the effects of death and dying

   c. spiritual differences among various ethnic groups

   d. sources of hope in people who are ill

5. Which of the following statements is NOT true of terminally ill patients?

   a. terminally ill patients have the same needs as any other patients

   b. terminally ill patients are frequently ignored by health care professionals, who are focused on prolonging life

   c. dying tends to produce feelings of isolation and fear in the patient

   d. terminally ill patients have an increasing need to know they are valued as human beings

6. Concerning attitudes toward death and dying in America, which one of the following statements is NOT true?

   a. acceptance of death as a natural process is still a difficult concept for most of the population to handle

   b. death is often seen by physicians as failure

   c. Americans continue to have death-denying attitudes, probably influenced by decreased exposure to death in the home, along with media and societal values extolling youth and health

   d. hospice staff should be able to remove the fears associated with dying

7. In hospice, the patient and family are considered the unit of care. Which statement most accurately describes dying patients and their families?

   a. a search for meaning and purpose in life is a common experience for dying patients and their families

   b. dying patients and their families are too consumed with financial problems ever to think about spiritual concerns

   c. dying patients and their families have little to fear because hospice takes care of everything

   d. the same care plan can be used for all families because their needs are the same

8. Which of the following situations can be felt by the dying patient as abandonment?

   (1) while the person is an inpatient on a medical floor, the doctor's visits are shorter and less frequent

   (2) a nurse assures the patient everything is going to be fine

   (3) a cousin tells the patient not to talk about dying because it is bad luck

   (4) the patient experiences ongoing pain because the doctor is concerned about addiction

   Choose the correct answer from the following:

   a. (1), (3), and (4)

   b. (3) and (4)

   c. (1), (2), and (3)

   d. all of the above

9. The modern hospice movement came about because dying patients' needs were neglected in acute care settings. As opposed to acute care, hospice focuses on:

   a. monitoring the disease process

   b. prolonging life

   c. comfort of the patient

   d. improvement of abnormal blood work

10. Hospice is:

   a. utilized when nothing more can be done

   b. a philosophy of care to improve quality of life for the terminally ill

   c. a place where people are sent to die

   d. available to patients and families on weekdays

# The Interdisciplinary Team

1. The successful hospice interdisciplinary team (IDT) views the role of each professional:

    a. as well defined and with specified boundaries

    b. to be carried out totally independent of other disciplines

    c. as reflecting unique expertise that is integrated into a coordinated team approach

    d. as one to be performed without personal involvement or emotional attachment

2. At regularly scheduled IDT meetings, all EXCEPT one of the following should be addressed as each care plan is reviewed:

    a. effectiveness of symptom management

    b. plan for telling the patient and family how to cope

    c. disease trajectory

    d. spiritual and psychosocial needs

3. According to experienced hospice professionals, the important qualities to look for in selecting hospice staff are:

    a. experience in care of the dying and sensitivity

    b. spirituality, hospice experience, and flexibility

    c. background in counseling and psychology

    d. flexibility, openness, and autonomy

4. To be an effective hospice IDT member, an individual should:

    a. express total resolution/acceptance of one's own death

    b. be open concerning one's own fears about death and be comfortable listening to other viewpoints

    c. have a definite belief in an afterlife and be able to explain that ideology to a patient

    d. be beyond all fear of death and expect that to be the ultimate goal of others

5. The use of volunteers in a Medicare-approved hospice:

   a. is a required component of the program

   b. is optional if there isn't a need for these services

   c. may be helpful in assisting the volunteers to resolve their personal grief

   d. is useful only if the volunteers have some background in caring for dying patients

6. Dietitians serve an important function as team members because they can:

   a. suggest interventions individualized to patients' food preferences and swallowing capacity

   b. suggest interventions for restoring good nutritional status

   c. suggest interventions for weight gain in emaciated patients

   d. suggest assessment parameters for all nutritional deficiencies

7. The chaplain or pastoral care person on the IDT is:

   a. always the bereavement coordinator

   b. expected to promote his or her own tenets of faith

   c. expected to be open to a wide range of values and beliefs

   d. responsible for assuring a peaceful death

8. The use of specialized consultants, such as physical therapists, occupational therapists, or psychologists:

   a. is not indicated for this population of patients

   b. is not indicated for most terminal patients, although all bedridden patients need physical therapy

   c. is not indicated because these consultants don't contribute to symptom management

   d. may greatly enhance quality of life by increasing mobility, independence, and meaningful activity

9. Staff support and team building will include the following activity:

    a. discouraging humor and laughing because they can be upsetting to the terminally ill patient

    b. encouraging team members to "keep it to themselves" when something is bothering them so negative thoughts don't get started

    c. letting nurses know it is inappropriate to cry when a patient dies

    d. avoiding discussion of specific personal problems or undermining self-esteem in group processes

10. Conflicts arise with any team of people who must work closely in intense situations. Principles of conflict resolution include:

    a. being prepared to defend your own position or point of view

    b. encouraging openness and creating a safe atmosphere for self-expression

    c. attacking the guilty person in the group meeting so the conflict can come to a quick resolution

    d. ignoring conflicts as long as possible; sooner or later everyone forgets about them

# Family Dynamics and Therapeutic Communication

1. In Jewish custom, the body of the deceased is never left alone because:

   a. of a lack of trust in health care providers

   b. doing so would show disrespect for the deceased

   c. if the body is left alone, the spirit may become angered and seek revenge

   d. none of the above

2. The family who has open communication, interdependence, and predictability are described as:

   a. an open family system

   b. an enmeshed family system

   c. a disengaged family system

   d. a differentiated family system

3. In the process of assessing the family system, interdisciplinary team members would do all of the following EXCEPT:

   a. diplomatically exclude the patient when discussing future plans

   b. accept each family member at his or her stage of development

   c. expect that the family will have a common history of family myths, secrets, and memories

   d. recognize that because relationships in a family are usually interdependent, it is best to work with the entire family

4. In looking at patient and family coping responses, you would expect:

   a. people who have regularly attended church not to have questions about meaning and purpose

   b. professional people, such as teachers or nurses, not to have dependency needs

   c. a degree of sadness to be present regardless of strong family support, good income, and religious faith

   d. each individual to fit into one of two coping responses, "closed" or "open"

5. Therapeutic dialogue includes active listening, empathy, and a nonjudgmental attitude. A good phrase to use is:

   a. "I understand what you are saying. This is how I would . . ."

   b. "Don't cry, everything is going to be OK."

   c. "The most important thing is . . ."

   d. "So, you feel . . . "

6. If a person of the Jewish faith dies while in the hospice program, you would expect the family to do all of the following EXCEPT:

   a. complete the grieving process at the end of 6 months

   b. refuse autopsy

   c. plan the burial within 24 hours

   d. use a plain casket

7. Therapeutic communication becomes reality through the following actions:

   a. sharing your personal experience so the other person has an example of the correct way to approach the problem

   b. conveying that you know exactly how the person is feeling

   c. scheduling a meeting to include the patient and family so they can jointly deal with information and engage in problem solving together

   d. making it clear that all hope is gone so the person can make realistic decisions

8. When the patient is in denial—for example, talking about future plans for recovery despite the fact that he or she has been clearly informed of the terminal stage of disease—you know that:

   a. the patient is a stubborn and unrealistic person

   b. denial is a method of coping, which the patient needs at this time

   c. it is your job to insist that the patient verbalize the truth

   d. everyone with terminal illness goes through denial, and reality will set in as the condition worsens

9. Hospice team members serve as facilitators to optimize the coping capacity of the patient and family members. The facilitator role includes:

   a. repeating or paraphrasing statements to encourage clarification of problems

   b. becoming deeply involved so the patient and family become dependent on you

   c. pointing out the most important problem the family should deal with first

   d. suggesting solutions to the family's problems

10. Hospice team members facilitate patient/family coping by taking all BUT one of the following actions:

    a. offering instruction in and support for caregiver skills indicated for the patient's comfort

    b. permitting the caregiver to provide needed assistance even though you could do it faster and more efficiently

    c. encouraging verbalization of fears and concerns

    d. not discussing any of the serious complications anticipated because it may be depressing

11. Some cultural differences to remember when caring for people of Chinese descent are that:

    a. they are stoic in the face of pain or bad news and are openly verbal about their illness and problems

    b. they believe in reincarnation but that they are powerless to influence what form their next life will take

    c. personal feelings, decisions, and interactions are kept within the family, with females having the dominant role

    d. they believe illness is an imbalance or disharmony within self, or as the self interacts with the environment, and they honor centuries-old methods of restoring balance

12. There are similarities in beliefs about life and death among most Native American tribes. All BUT one of the following are generally observed:

    a. they accept death as a natural and expected event

    b. the body is respected, and cremation is not usually done

    c. funeral rituals are brief and confined to the immediate family

    d. a remembrance is kept as a reminder to strive for virtuous behavior during the year of mourning

# Disease Processes Common to Hospice

1. The patient's level of physical ability and function is a key to prognostication in terminal disease. This level is best documented by:

   a. a Karnofsky Performance Status Scale

   b. vital signs

   c. muscle-strength testing by a physical therapist

   d.  weight and protein intake

2. The AIDS virus primarily affects T-lymphocytes and has a high affinity to which specific cell?

   a. macrophages

   b. HIV

   c. CD4

   d. eosinophils

3. The most frequently occurring malignancy in persons with AIDS is:

   a. lung cancer

   b. tuberculosis

   c. Kaposi's sarcoma

   d. myeloma

4. Because the AIDS virus causes serious suppression of the immune system, patients are highly susceptible to opportunistic infections, the most common of which is:

   a. pseudomonas

   b. PCP (*Pneumocystis carinii* pneumonia)

   c. tuberculosis

   d. disseminated CMV (cytomegalovirus)

5. The preferred treatment regimen for *Pneumocystis carinii* pneumonia is:

   a. isoniazid (INH)

   b. amphotericin (Amphotericin-B)

   c. fluconazole (Diflucan)

   d. trimethoprim-sulfamethoxazole (TMP-SMZ, Bactrim, Septra)

6. Which cancer treatment modality is a systemic treatment and results in systemic side effects?

   a. surgery

   b. intravenous or oral chemotherapy

   c. radiation implants

   d. external beam radiation

7. The side effect of chemotherapy most frequently of concern to patients is:

   a. neurotoxicity—peripheral neuropathies, constipation

   b. nephrotoxicity—blood in urine, renal failure

   c. gastrointestinal symptoms—nausea, vomiting, diarrhea

   d. cardiotoxicity—loss of cardiac muscle tone, congestive heart failure

8. Which side effect of chemotherapy can be asymptomatic but has serious life-threatening potential?

   a. bone marrow suppression—especially the white cells, making the patient susceptible to infections

   b. epithelial denudement of the gastrointestinal tract

   c. bone marrow suppression—especially the red cells, making the patient susceptible to anemia

   d. anorexia and weight loss

9. Caregivers taking care of a patient with AIDS in the home should be given the following instructions:

   (1) gloves should be worn when handling any body fluids

   (2) gloves do not need to be worn for routine bathing if there are no open wounds or incontinence

   (3) dishes and utensils used by the patient should be washed separately

   (4) unless there is a bathroom that can be used solely by the patient, the patient should use a bedside commode

   Choose the correct answer from the following:

   a. (1) and (2)

   b. (1), (2), and (3)

   c. (1) and (3)

   d. all of the above

10. Medications that can color urine, feces, sputum, sweat, and tears a red-orange color and stain soft contact lenses are:

    a. dapsone (Aviosulfon) and pentamidine (Nebupent)

    b. isoniazid (INH) and ethambutol (Myambutol)

    c. rifabutin (Mycobutin) and rifampin (Rifadin)

    d. azithromycin (Zithromax) and clarithromycin (Biaxin)

11. The last function to exhibit signs and symptoms of failure in amyotrophic lateral sclerosis (ALS) would be:

    a. speech

    b. swallowing

    c. walking

    d. mental faculties

12. A trial of gamma globulin or corticosteroids may be used when the patient has a diagnosis of:

    a. cerebrovascular accident

    b. amyotrophic lateral sclerosis (ALS)

    c. multiple sclerosis (MS)

    d. Parkinson's disease

13. Which of the following is associated with the highest mortality risk?

    a. acute liver failure associated with alcoholic cirrhosis over 1 week

    b. three different organ systems in failure over 3 days

    c. heart failure symptoms lasting more than 2 weeks

    d. renal crisis with fluid and electrolyte imbalance, with BUN remaining abnormal after 5 days of treatment

14. In the second edition of the National Hospice Organization's *Medical Guidelines for Determining Prognosis in Selected Non-Cancer Diseases,* all EXCEPT one of the following are listed under general guidelines for limited prognosis regardless of diagnosis:

    a. hemoglobin less than 5

    b. recent functional status decline to less than 50% on the Karnofsky Performance Status Scale

    c. unintentional progressive weight loss of more than 10% over the previous 6 months

    d. a life-limiting disease with documented clinical progression

15. The most commonly occurring oncologic emergency is:

    a. pleural effusion

    b. bowel obstruction

    c. hypercalcemia

    d. superior vena cava syndrome

# Imminent Death

1. A purplish or blotchy red-blue coloring, also called mottling, usually begins on the knees or feet and progresses to the entire lower extremity. This is a sign that:

   a. the patient is in need of cardiac stimulation

   b. electric blankets need to be applied to prevent chills

   c. the patient is near death and no intervention is likely to reverse the symptom

   d. the patient's legs should be massaged and/or placed lower than the torso to improve circulation

2. One indication of approaching death is change in the circulatory system, evidenced by the following changes in blood pressure and heart rate:

   a. decreasing blood pressure and increasing heart rate (but weaker)

   b. decreasing blood pressure and decreasing heart rate (but stronger)

   c. increasing blood pressure and increasing heart rate (but weaker)

   d. increasing blood pressure and decreasing heart rate (but stronger)

3. During "active dying," the last days and hours, the senses may be overactive or underactive. If the dying person's senses are overactive, one should:

   a. talk louder so the person will know someone is present

   b. provide lots of activity and lively music

   c. administer large doses of muscle relaxants

   d. reduce external stimuli

4. A buildup of secretions in the upper-respiratory tract, causing what is sometimes called the "death rattle," can be managed by the following:

> (1) decreasing fluid intake
>
> (2) frequent repositioning
>
> (3) keeping the head of the bed in a raised position
>
> (4) administering medications such as anticholinergics

Choose the correct answer from the following:

a. (2), (3), and (4)

b. (2) and (4)

c. (3) and (4)

d. all of the above

5. In the last days or hours of life, evidences of body shutdown will include all of the following EXCEPT:

a. breathing may change in rate, depth, and rhythm

b. hearing will be the first of the sensory functions to fail

c. urine will become darker in color with diminished output

d. bowel and bladder incontinence will occur as sphincter muscles relax

6. The family will benefit from guidance and support from team members to be reassured that they are doing the right thing and that their actions are comforting to the patient. Which of the following would NOT be one of your suggestions to them:

a. don't talk directly to an unresponsive patient because it would be insulting

b. anticipate the needs of the patient

c. continue to explain your actions prior to care procedures

d. watch for nonverbal signs of discomfort such as moaning or restlessness

7.  The family should be prepared for changes in the patient's physical appearance as death nears. This will include:

    a. puffy eyes and cheeks

    b. clenched jaw

    c. pale, bluish or grayish skin

    d. earlobes may fall forward, away from the cranium

8.  Patients who are imminently dying usually exhibit dependent edema as a result of:

    a. increased metabolism

    b. increased circulatory proteins

    c. increased activity

    d. increased heart failure

9.  Respiratory changes in the last days or hours—such as Cheyne Stokes respirations, dyspnea, or obvious rales—are caused by:

    (1) metabolic imbalance

    (2) tumor or fluid in the lungs

    (3) poor cardiac functioning

    (4) inefficient oxygen perfusion

    Choose the correct answer from the following:

    a. (1) and (2)

    b. (3) and (4)

    c. (2), (3), and (4)

    d. all of the above

10. When a family member reports that the patient is "seeing" his dead mother, you would respond in the following way:

    a. ask the patient, "What was it like?"

    b. explain to the patient why this is impossible

    c. suggest sedation

    d. restrain the patient to prevent self-injury

# Concepts of Grief and Bereavement

1. The definition of *grief* is:

   a. the cultural response to having suffered a loss

   b. the process of psychological, social, and somatic reactions to a perceived loss

   c. the state of having suffered a loss

   d. the process of psychological, social, and somatic reactions to a perceived future loss

2. The definition of *anticipatory grief* is:

   a. the cultural response to having suffered a loss

   b. the process of psychological, social, and somatic reactions to a perceived loss

   c. the state of having suffered a loss

   d. the process of psychological, social, and somatic reactions to a perceived future loss

3. The definition of *mourning* is:

   a. the cultural response to having suffered a loss

   b. the process of psychological, social, and somatic reactions to a perceived loss

   c. the state of having suffered a loss

   d. the process of psychological, social, and somatic reactions to a perceived future loss

4. The definition of *bereavement* is:

   a. the cultural response to having suffered a loss

   b. the process of psychological, social, and somatic reactions to a perceived loss

   c. the state of having suffered a loss

   d. the process of psychological, social, and somatic reactions to a perceived future loss

5. According to Worden, the first task of grief resolution is:

   a. to take care of the legal things as soon as possible

   b. to plan a meaningful funeral service

   c. to accept the reality of the loss

   d. to get rid of the deceased's belongings so there aren't so many reminders around

6. If you make a follow-up bereavement call, and the widow tells you she can't seem to concentrate on anything, is not sleeping well, and when she does sleep she has vivid dreams of the deceased—sometimes even hears him speaking to her during the day—your response would be:

   a. "Have you ever had a problem like this before?"

   b. "Would you like me to make an appointment for our psychiatrist to visit you?"

   c. "Did you take a sleeping pill? Sometimes that causes strange dreams."

   d. "These are all normal reactions, experienced by many people."

7. The extent and duration of grief:

   a. vary considerably from person to person

   b. differ considerably between men and women

   c. are the same when death is expected and planned for

   d. are pretty much the same for everyone

8. For grief to be pathological, it must be:

   a. more than a year in duration

   b. affecting all aspects of the person's life

   c. preceded by depression

   d. none of the above—grief cannot be pathological

9. According to Worden, one of the principles of grief counseling is to help the survivor to actualize the loss. One of the most important ways in which we can accomplish this is:

    a. to encourage the survivor to speak only of positive things

    b. to permit the survivor to repeat the story of the death event as many times as he or she wishes

    c. after several tellings of the story of the death, to try to change the conversation

    d. to encourage talk about plans for the future instead of dwelling on the past

10. When we see a widow who has complicated or pathological mourning, we should make a referral for more intense counseling than the hospice team is prepared to provide. The signs of this include all of the following EXCEPT:

    a. inability to experience typical emotional reactions to loss

    b. severe deterioration of functional status

    c. "overactivity" to avoid feelings

    d. patterns of self-destructive behaviors or relationships

# Spiritual Care

1. Spiritual care of the hospice patient and family:

    a. is provided in accordance with the religion of the hospice chaplain

    b. is provided only by a hospice staff member

    c. is provided to every single patient and family admitted to hospice care

    d. identifies and strives to relieve the spiritual suffering of the patient and family

2. Spiritual comfort is most appropriately provided to the hospice patient in the following way:

    a. making sure prayers are said at the bedside every day

    b. encouraging the patient to make his or her peace with God

    c. offering the patient tapes of your favorite hymns

    d. being present and listening for expressions of spiritual distress

3. The spiritual part of human life refers to the inner self and its relationship to all BUT one of the following:

    a. a higher power

    b. church rituals

    c. other people in one's life

    d. the universe

4. The religious part of human life refers to all BUT one of the following:

    a. anointing

    b. doing penance

    c. seeking reconciliation

    d. receiving the sacrament of communion

5. Listening as a patient engages in life review:

   a. could have a negative impact if it includes unpleasant things

   b. should not be done because it will be personal and private information

   c. would encourage something that is a waste of precious time

   d. can help the patient identify values and spiritual pains

6. Spiritual needs concerning such matters as meaning of life and suffering, forgiveness, and belonging are frequently seen in dying patients. They are generally referred to as "universal spiritual needs" because:

   a. they appear to be present in most people, regardless of their culture or religion

   b. they are true for all Christians around the globe

   c. they are the ultimate quests of spiritualism

   d. they need to be addressed whether the patient wants to or not

7. Treatment strategies for spiritual suffering may include all BUT one of the following:

   a. reading scriptures

   b. sitting with the patient

   c. encouraging the patient to think only of pleasant things

   d. providing music desired by the patient

8. Spiritual need is one piece of a holistic assessment that should:

   a. include what is meaningful or frightening to the patient

   b. always be done by the hospice chaplain

   c. fully describe the rules of the church the patient attends

   d. never be discussed on the first visit

9. When assessing the patient and family for spiritual needs, you will find:

   a. consistency in beliefs within the same family

   b. that it requires going beyond your personal ideas of right and wrong

   c. that if the patient or family members don't bring up the subject, there are likely no problems

   d. that the family members will always share their inner pain, but the patient seldom does

10. Inner anguish, or spiritual distress, may be caused by:

   a. guilt because of past wrongdoings

   b. feeling alienated from God

   c. being afraid to die

   d. all of the above

# Pain Management

1. Pain is:

    a. easily and objectively identified by the nurse

    b. whatever the patient says it is

    c. always preventable if detected early enough

    d. something that must be endured to avoid addiction

2. Which of the following pain medications must not be crushed?

    a. morphine sulfate SR (Contin, Oramorph)

    b. acetaminophen (Tylenol) with codeine

    c. Percocet/Percodan

    d. hydromorphone (Dilaudid)

3. A "ceiling dose" of a medication is:

    a. the maximum dose giving therapeutic results without undesirable side effects

    b. the maximum safe dose to prevent respiratory depression

    c. the highest dose the pharmacy will dispense

    d. the highest dose in which the drug is manufactured

4. The "ceiling dose" of acetaminophen (Tylenol) is:

    a. 500 mg every 24 hours

    b. 6,000 mg every 24 hours

    c. 4,000 mg every 24 hours

    d. unlimited

5. Patients taking narcotics on a regular schedule must:

    a. wake themselves at night to prevent respiratory depression

    b. adjust the amount of medication they use depending on the time of day

    c. plan to wean themselves off narcotics as soon as possible

    d. be placed on a daily bowel regimen to prevent constipation

6. The two most common barriers to pain control are:

    a. deceit and lying

    b. fear and ignorance

    c. hopelessness and silence

    d. mistrust and malpractice

7. Bone pain is usually characterized by:

    a. a dull, steady, "aching" sensation

    b. a "burning" sensation

    c. predictable waves of pain

    d. colicky, stabbing pain

8. Neuropathic pain is often characterized by:

    a. a dull, steady, "aching" sensation

    b. a "burning" sensation

    c. predictable waves of pain

    d. colicky, stabbing pain

9. Antidepressants or anticonvulsants have specific action on:

    a. neuropathic pain

    b. bone pain

    c. visceral pain

    d. abdominal pain

10. Nonsteroidal anti-inflammatory drugs (NSAIDs) may be used alone or with narcotics, specifically for:

    a. neuropathic pain

    b. bone pain

    c. visceral pain

    d. abdominal pain

11. For the patient with persistent pain from metastatic cancer, pain medications should be given:

    a. PRN to avoid addiction and tolerance

    b. four times daily

    c. via a patch or intravenously for more severe pain

    d. around the clock on a regular schedule, plus a PRN dose for "breakthrough" pain

12. Why are phenothiazines commonly used as narcotic adjuvants for chronic pain?

    a. antianxiety activity

    b. antiemetic activity

    c. analgesic activity

    d. *a* and *b* above

13. For patients placed on SR (sustained-release) narcotics for chronic pain relief, which of the following drugs would be an appropriate choice for acute "breakthrough" pain?

    a. pentazocine (Talwin)

    b. hydromorphone (Dilaudid)

    c. butorphanol (Stadol)

    d. nalbuphine (Nubain)

14. Mr. S. rates his pain as 2 to 4 (on the 0- to 10-point pain scale) but insists on the need for stronger medication (a narcotic) or some new plan to relieve his pain. The basis for your response is:

    a. that pain at 2 does not require further intervention

    b. that Mr. S. is being unrealistic in expecting total relief

    c. that Mr. S.'s lack of willingness to tolerate pain at 2 directs the plan

    d. that the risks of narcotic use are not warranted in this situation

15. Which of the following narcotic analgesics is usually NOT preferred in chronic pain due to the drug's short duration of action?

    a. meperidine (Demerol)

    b. morphine

    c. aspirin

    d. methadone

16. When a patient begins on opioids, he or she may experience a number of side effects, but in time these will usually decrease as tolerance is developed. The one side effect that always continues to be a problem is:

    a. respiratory depression

    b. nausea and vomiting

    c. constipation

    d. drowsiness

17. Neuritic-type pains, which the patient might describe as burning or shooting, would best be treated with which type of drug?

    a. opioid

    b. nonsteroidal anti-inflammatory drug (NSAID)

    c. tricyclic antidepressant

    d. skeletal muscle relaxant

18. If the patient has a brain tumor and headache that may be caused from edema around the tumor, a useful medication to add to the current analgesic regime would be:

    a. dexamethasone (Decadron)

    b. phenobarbital

    c. hydrochlorothiazide (HydroDiuril)

    d. acetaminophen (Tylenol)

19. If a patient is on morphine sulfate 20 mg four times per day and states that it gives good pain relief but that the relief only lasts for 3 hours and the pain always returns before time for the next dose, the following should be considered:

    a. change the morphine sulfate dose to every 3 hours

    b. increase the dose of morphine sulfate

    c. change to a different analgesic

    d. add diazepam (Valium) to relax the patient

20. The fentanyl transdermal (Duragesic) patch is subcutaneously absorbed analgesia and:

    a. is routinely changed every 72 hours

    b. absorbs better on skin over some adipose or muscle tissue

    c. can be changed every 48 hours if the patient consistently has increased pain on the third day

    d. all of the above

# Symptom Control

1. Mr. J. has severe stomatitis and esophagitis. Appropriate intervention would include:

   a. clear liquid diet

   b. lemon-glycerin swab PRN

   c. nonsteroidal anti-inflammatory drugs (NSAIDs)

   d. viscous lidocaine (Xylocaine) 2% by mouth every 2 to 3 hours PRN

2. The drug of choice for treating an active seizure is:

   a. diazepam (Valium)

   b. amitriptyline (Elavil)

   c. prochlorperazine (Compazine)

   d. prednisone

3. Intractable hiccups may be best treated with:

   a. ondansetron (Zofran)

   b. phenytoin (Dilantin)

   c. megesterol (Megace)

   d. chlorpromazine (Thorazine)

4. Dyspnea, in a patient with lung cancer, is best treated with:

   a. oxygen by nasal cannula

   b. low-dose morphine

   c. theophylline

   d. aminophylline

5. Almost all patients with advanced cancer experience progressive generalized weakness. Strength can be restored by the following:

   a. blood transfusion

   b. medications such as megesterol (Megace)

   c. steroids

   d. none of the above

6. The most appropriate drug for confusion and agitation is:

    a. prochlorperazine (Compazine)

    b. morphine sulfate

    c. haloperidol (Haldol)

    d. dexamethasone (Decadron)

7. About 20% of terminally ill patients develop ankle edema. The nurse would do all EXCEPT one of the following:

    a. encourage exercise, especially walking

    b. consider stopping or changing drugs causing fluid retention

    c. encourage fluids to keep the kidneys working

    d. suggest full-length compression stockings

8. Mrs. L. is admitted with end-stage cancer, and one of her problems is syncope. Which of the following should be done?

    a. consider discontinuing antihypertensive medications if blood pressure is consistently low

    b. encourage her to remain in bed

    c. encourage her to drink less fluid to avoid needing to go to the bathroom

    d. restrain her in bed so she can't fall

9. The use of morphine in patients with lung cancer who suffer from exertional dyspnea:

    a. is dangerous because it reduces respirations

    b. is totally inappropriate because it will lead to addiction

    c. reduces tachypnea and overventilation, making breathing more efficient

    d. is a bad choice as the dose will gradually need to be increased

10. A cough that prevents sleep and rest can usually be effectively palliated by:

    a. dry air

    b. a codeine preparation

    c. sour or spicy foods

    d. suppressing expectorations

11. All EXCEPT one of the following drugs are indicated to control nausea:

    a. prochlorperazine (Compazine)

    b. dextroamphetamine (Dexedrine)

    c. haloperidol (Haldol)

    d. metoclopramide (Reglan)

12. Anorexia and resulting cachexia contribute to weakness, decreased activity, and depression. When megesterol (Megace) is prescribed to increase appetite:

    a. it is very effective and inexpensive

    b. there are no side effects to be concerned about

    c. cachexia is reversed dramatically

    d. in large doses (400 to 800 mg daily), some patients note temporary improvement

13. Decreased mobility and activity, decreased intake, and analgesics all contribute to the problem of constipation frequently observed in terminal patients. All EXCEPT one of the following are appropriate interventions:

    a. give psyllium (Metamucil) as a laxative when the patient has limited intake

    b. place all patients who are inactive and on routine analgesics on a regular bowel protocol

    c. urge increased liquids and dietary roughage

    d. increase mobility

14. On a home visit, Mrs. R., who has a primary cancer of the liver, complains that she has been bothered by diarrhea for the past 2 days, having had six to seven very loose stools per day. All of the following actions should be considered EXCEPT:

    a. obtain an order for pancreatic enzymes

    b. advise patient to decrease oral intake

    c. check for impaction

    d. obtain an order for loperamide (Imodium)

15. Mechanical debridement by saline wet-to-dry dressing or a hydrocolloidal dressing might be used for skin breakdown in:

    a. Stage I

    b. Stage II

    c. Stage III

    d. Stage IV

16. Mr. T. has end-stage colon cancer with advanced liver metastases, resulting in jaundice and pruritis. These symptoms can be relieved by all EXCEPT:

    a. topical creams

    b. a very hot bath

    c. medications such as hydroxyzine (Atarax) or diphenhydramine (Benadryl)

    d. cholestyramine (Questran, Cholybar) 4 g every 6 to 8 hours, reducing bile salt absorption

17. It is inappropriate to plan aggressive curative treatment when:

    a. cure is possible

    b. there is a realistic chance of worthwhile prolongation of life

    c. the side effects of the treatment are more distressing than the potential benefits

    d. a patient chooses a clinical trial with informed consent

18. An appropriate criterion for deciding to institute any given therapy for a terminally ill patient is:

    a. if the potential benefits outweigh the potential risks or burdens to the patient

    b. if the physician wants to try once more for a cure

    c. if the family demands it

    d. if it will prolong life

# Palliative Nutrition and Hydration

1. *Palliative nutrition* means:

   a. providing whatever the patient desires for comfort

   b. providing sufficient protein, calories, and fat to regain optimal nutrition

   c. providing a low-sodium diet to prevent edema

   d. providing artificial feeding so the patient won't suffer from starvation

2. The fact that patients with advanced disease and multisystem failure do not suffer discomfort from dehydration is likely because:

   a. it is usually eunatremic dehydration (neither hypernatremia nor hyponatremia)

   b. it is a state that develops gradually

   c. it is a natural course when the body is "shutting down"

   d. all of the above

   e. none of the above

3. The Supreme Court in the Cruzan case voiced an opinion that artificial nutrition and hydration:

   a. are not medical treatments and cannot be refused

   b. should always be administered

   c. are always in the patient's best interest

   d. can be refused just as any other medical treatment

4. Artificial nutrition and hydration should be used in terminally ill patients with inadequate intake:

   a. to improve their strength

   b. only in very rare cases where a bona fide benefit can be realized

   c. to improve their nutritional status

   d. to ensure adequate intake of proteins, fats, and carbohydrates

5. Artificially provided fluids for nutrition or hydration in a patient with end-stage disease and multisystem failure are:

   a. usually not beneficial due to inefficient physiologic and metabolic processes

   b. beneficial to increase comfort

   c. useful in decreasing the extracellular fluids

   d. known to prolong life

6. Studies have shown that patients who are terminally ill and have limited intake are usually comfortable despite varying degrees of dehydration. One of the theories about why this may occur is that:

   a. electrolyte imbalance is common

   b. patients are hyponatremic instead of hypernatremic

   c. dynorphin production is increased

   d. patients suddenly reduce their intake

7. A patient with a head and neck cancer who has had high doses of radiation therapy to the neck area is likely to have a dry and inflamed oral cavity. The therapeutic approach would be to:

   a. provide salt water rinses

   b. increase moisture content of foods

   c. provide hot but soft foods

   d. limit the use of artificial saliva because of its mineral content

8. If a patient is not eating because of nausea, the following action may help the problem:

   a. avoid all medications around mealtime

   b. offer mildly flavored foods in small servings

   c. encourage exercise after eating

   d. encourage the patient to be in the kitchen while the meal is being prepared

9. Discussions and printed material should be shared with family and friends to help them understand the changing nutritional needs of the patient. The following information should be included:

   a. since a cancer utilizes calories and nutrients, the intake must be increased

   b. the family can force the patient to eat more easily than a nurse can because they can use guilt tactics

   c. the experience of eating is no longer a pleasure for the patient

   d. fluids should be pushed in every way possible

10. Providing artificial nutrition and hydration to terminal patients who are dehydrated and malnourished:

    a. has the potential for more complications than benefits

    b. is a good way to show professional concern and caring

    c. proves the patient is not being abandoned

    d. is an effective way of improving the patient's performance status

# Legal and Ethical Issues

1. In 1991, the Patient Self-Determination Act (PSDA) was passed as part of Medicare legislation. Identify one statement in the following list that is NOT true of the PSDA.

   a. only agencies that are reimbursed by Medicare must comply

   b. the PSDA requires the patient to have an advance directive before admission to a health care facility

   c. the PSDA requires the agency to ask a patient upon admission if there is an advance directive

   d. when there is an advance directive, the agency must make it part of the patient's record and honor it

2. Which of the following is true about advance directives?

   a. Pennsylvania was one of the first states to have pertinent legislation

   b. a person doesn't need a "living will" if he or she already has a will

   c. living wills must be done by a lawyer and notarized

   d. living wills, durable power of attorney for health care, and treatment preferences are all examples of advance directives

3. A person who is terminally ill has the right to know the truth about his or her condition, prognosis, and options. The exception to this is:

   a. when the family asks you not to, knowing the patient "can't take it"

   b. when the doctor feels it would have a negative impact

   c. when the patient requests not to talk about it

   d. when the nurse feels doing so would cause depression

4. Most patients have an advance directive requesting that no more curative or aggressive measures be performed if they have a terminal illness. However, we cannot assume that every patient wishes to decline certain procedures, such as cardiopulmonary resuscitation (CPR). Which of the following is true about hospice and CPR?

    a. hospice consent may include an acknowledgment that CPR will not be provided by the hospice team

    b. the patient must have do-not-resuscitate (DNR) status to enter hospice

    c. if the patient requests CPR, hospice staff must perform this

    d. if the patient doesn't have an advance directive, it's obvious he or she doesn't want to talk about it

5. It is only in recent years that state governments have passed laws permitting registered nurses to have any part in death pronouncement. The following statement is true:

    a. state laws vary, and counties within each state may have different protocols on who should contact whom

    b. every state permits R.N.'s to pronounce the death if they know the patient and have been providing care

    c. only a doctor can determine that a patient is dead

    d. the coroner is always notified when a patient dies outside a hospital

6. Ethical principles include autonomy, beneficence, justice, veracity, and nonmaleficence. These principles have evolved from the study of ethics, which refers to:

    a. psychological thought

    b. community benefactors

    c. moral issues

    d. determining right and wrong

7. Select the correct definition of *beneficence*.

    a. truth telling, not deceiving

    b. right to self-determination

    c. equal access to care without discrimination

    d. doing good, acting in the patient's best interest

8. Select the correct definition of *autonomy.*

   a. truth telling, not deceiving

   b. right to self-determination

   c. equal access to care without discrimination

   d. doing good, acting in the patient's best interest

9. Select the correct definition of *veracity.*

   a. truth telling, not deceiving

   b. right to self-determination

   c. equal access to care without discrimination

   d. doing good, acting in the patient's best interest

10. Some ethical dilemmas have straightforward decision paths, such as which one of the following:

   a. if the patient and family are disagreeing, it is up to the doctor to decide the course of action

   b. if the patient and family are disagreeing, the patient's wishes should be followed

   c. if the patient and family are disagreeing, always take the family's side because that's who will be around to sue you later

   d. if the patient and family are disagreeing, tell them you'll be back when they've worked it out

# Continuity of Care
## and the Medicare Hospice Benefit

1. When the total cumulative care days of all patients in your hospice program are added up, the ratio of home care to inpatient care must be:

   a. 50% home, 50% inpatient

   b. 60% home, 40% inpatient

   c. 80% home, 20% inpatient

   d. 20% home, 80% inpatient

2. Before choosing the Medicare Hospice Benefit, patients need information about the benefit. Which of the following is NOT true?

   a. they may select any hospice program they wish

   b. hospice focuses on care and comfort, not cure

   c. Social Security payments are not affected

   d. there may be a small charge for prescription drugs

3. Before signing the Medicare Hospice Benefit election form, patients should be informed that they:

   a. will now receive care for all conditions from hospice staff

   b. will receive comprehensive care from an interdisciplinary team for their incurable condition

   c. must first get permission to continue curative treatments for the terminal illness

   d. must pay for rental of any medical equipment they need, such as a hospital bed or wheelchair

4. If the patient decides to revoke the Medicare Hospice Benefit, the patient and family need to know that:

   a. their current certification remains valid if they choose to come back later

   b. they will lose the remaining days of the current period

   c. they can come back anytime and pick up where they left off

   d. once they leave the program, they cannot come back

5. At the beginning of each benefit period, the patient must be "certified" by a physician. This means:

    a. the patient is known to be eligible for Medicare

    b. the patient is competent to make his or her own decisions

    c. the patient no longer has insurance coverage for hospitalization

    d. the patient has a terminal illness and a life expectancy of 6 months or less

6. The "core services" that must be provided by the hospice agency (not subcontracted) are:

    a. nurse, physician, volunteers

    b. social worker, nurse, home health aide

    c. nurse, social worker, counselor

    d. volunteers, nurse, social worker

7. The Medicare hospice manual describes all EXCEPT one of the following:

    a. program requirements to be Medicare approved

    b. hospice levels of care

    c. eligibility for the Medicare Hospice Benefit

    d. ideas for fundraising

8. If a Veterans Administration (VA) medical center has its own hospice program, it can be assumed that:

    a. it is automatically Medicare approved, being a federal agency

    b. it cannot collect Medicare reimbursement

    c. the program will be comprehensive, mandated from VA headquarters

    d. it is reimbursed by Medicare but must go through the same approval evaluation as any other hospice

9. Billing for the Medicare Hospice Benefit is sent to:

    a. a designated intermediary

    b. the Health Care Financing Administration (HCFA)

    c. the Medicare office in Washington

    d. individual hospice alliances or networks

10. Liaisons with physicians, community agencies, and health care facilities are necessary for providing continuity of care for hospice patients. *Liaison* means:

    a. letter of introduction

    b. the official person in your agency who can sign documents

    c. the person who sets the rules for exchanging information

    d. communication to ensure concerted and cooperative actions

# APPENDIX B

# Test Answers

## Chapter 1
### Hospice Philosophy

| | |
|---|---|
| 1. c | 6. d |
| 2. d | 7. a |
| 3. b | 8. d |
| 4. b | 9. c |
| 5. a | 10. b |

## Chapter 2
### Interdisciplinary Team

| | |
|---|---|
| 1. c | 6. a |
| 2. b | 7. c |
| 3. d | 8. d |
| 4. b | 9. d |
| 5. a | 10. b |

## Chapter 3
### Family Dynamics

| | |
|---|---|
| 1. b | 7. c |
| 2. a | 8. b |
| 3. a | 9. a |
| 4. c | 10. d |
| 5. d | 11. d |
| 6. a | 12. c |

## Chapter 4
### Disease Processes

| | |
|---|---|
| 1. a | 9. a |
| 2. c | 10. c |
| 3. c | 11. d |
| 4. b | 12. c |
| 5. d | 13. b |
| 6. b | 14. a |
| 7. c | 15. c |
| 8. a | |

## Chapter 5
### Imminent Death

| | |
|---|---|
| 1. c | 6. a |
| 2. a | 7. c |
| 3. d | 8. d |
| 4. d | 9. b |
| 5. b | 10. a |

## Chapter 6
### Grief and Bereavement

| | |
|---|---|
| 1. b | 6. d |
| 2. d | 7. a |
| 3. a | 8. b |
| 4. c | 9. b |
| 5. c | 10. c |

## Chapter 7
### Spiritual Care

| | | | |
|---|---|---|---|
| 1. d | | 6. a | |
| 2. d | | 7. c | |
| 3. b | | 8. a | |
| 4. c | | 9. b | |
| 5. d | | 10. d | |

## Chapter 8
### Pain Management

| | | | |
|---|---|---|---|
| 1. b | | 11. d | |
| 2. a | | 12. d | |
| 3. a | | 13. b | |
| 4. c | | 14. c | |
| 5. d | | 15. a | |
| 6. b | | 16. c | |
| 7. a | | 17. c | |
| 8. b | | 18. a | |
| 9. a | | 19. a | |
| 10. b | | 20. d | |

## Chapter 9
### Symptom Control

| | | | |
|---|---|---|---|
| 1. d | | 10. b | |
| 2. a | | 11. b | |
| 3. d | | 12. d | |
| 4. b | | 13. a | |
| 5. d | | 14. b | |
| 6. c | | 15. c | |
| 7. c | | 16. b | |
| 8. a | | 17. c | |
| 9. c | | 18. a | |

## Chapter 10
### Palliative Nutrition and Hydration

| | | | |
|---|---|---|---|
| 1. a | | 6. c | |
| 2. d | | 7. b | |
| 3. d | | 8. b | |
| 4. b | | 9. c | |
| 5. a | | 10. a | |

## Chapter 11
### Legal and Ethical Issues

| | | | |
|---|---|---|---|
| 1. b | | 6. c | |
| 2. d | | 7. d | |
| 3. c | | 8. b | |
| 4. a | | 9. a | |
| 5. a | | 10. b | |

## Chapter 12
### Continuity of Care and Medicare

| | | | |
|---|---|---|---|
| 1. c | | 6. c | |
| 2. a | | 7. d | |
| 3. b | | 8. b | |
| 4. b | | 9. a | |
| 5. d | | 10. d | |

# Index

Narcotics. *See* Analgesics
National Hospice Organization, xiii, 3,
    4, 15, 45, 91, 96, 196
Native American beliefs about death, 34
Nausea, 152–153, 173
Near-death experience, 65, 73–74
Needs of dying patients, 7–8, 96–99
Neurological disorders, 58–59
Neuropathic pain, 109, 110
*New Meanings of Death*, 6
NHO. *See* National Hospice
    Organization
Nociceptive pain, 109
Nurse practice acts, 187
Nurses, 19
Nutrition, 170–179
    artificial, 174–179
    and patient comfort, 170, 173
    teaching family about, 172, 174

O'Connor, Sandra Day, 176, 182
Odynophagia, 144
Oncologic emergencies, 154–155
*On Death and Dying*, 5
Open family system, 28
Opioids. *See* Analgesics
Organ system failure, 45
OSF, 45
*Overextended and Undernourished*, 24
*Oxford Textbook of Palliative Medicine*,
    xi, 10

Pain, 11–12, 14, 32, 103–120, 172
    assessment of, 109–111
    definition of, 104
    multiple causes of, 104–106
    origins of, 109
    terms relating to, 105
    treatments for, 111–120
    types of, 108
Painkillers. *See* Analgesics
Pain management, 109–120
    with adjuvant drugs, 116–117, 118
    barriers to, 108
    and calculating breakthrough
        dose, 116
    and changing drugs, 113, 116
    choosing drugs for, 112–113
    myth versus reality of, 106–107
    nonpharmacologic measures for,
        117, 119
    World Health Organization
        approach to, 111–112

Palliative care. *See also* Hospice;
    Hospice care
    application of, 11–15
    versus curative care, 8–10
    and patient comfort, 14–15, 170,
        173, 176–177
    transition to, 10–11
Parenteral hydration, 172
Paresthesia, 105
Parkes, Colin Murray, xiii, 8–9, 84
Parkes and Weiss's tasks for grief
    recovery, 85
Parkes' phases of mourning, 85
Parkinson's disease, 58
Patient rights, 183–187
Patient Self-Determination Act, 183
Performance scales, parameters of, 46
Performance status, 44–45
Pharmacists, 20
Physical appearance, at the end of life,
    65–66
Physician-assisted suicide, 189–190
Physicians, 19, 195
Pleural effusion, 146–147
*Pneumocystis carinii* pneumonia, 54
Portenoy, R. K., 107
Portnoy, Dennis, 24
President's Commission for the Study of
    Ethical Problems in Medicine
    and Biomedical and Behavioral
    Research, 176, 182
Pressure ulcers, 158
Prognosis, xiii, 45–47
Pruritis, 156
Pseudoaddiction, 105
Psychiatrists, 20
Psychologists, 20
Pulmonary failure, 56

Quint, Jeanne, 6

Radiation side effects, 50–51, 160, 164
Rahe, R. H., 82
Rando, Therese A., 78, 84, 88
Rando's six "R" processes of mourning,
    85
Reactive depression, 138
Relationships, with family, 28–29
Religious beliefs, 32–34
Religious needs, 96–97. *See also*
        Spiritual *terms*; Spirituality
Renal failure, 60
Rescue dose, 116

# About the Author

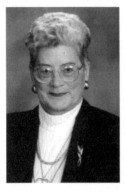

Shirley Ann Smith, R.N., M.S.N., C.R.N.H., is a graduate of Los Angeles County General Hospital/University of Southern California School of Nursing, Bloomsburg University, and the University of Pennsylvania. Her postgraduate studies include courses in medical ethics at College Misericordia and the University of Connecticut, as well as hospice studies at Kings College, London, England. She is a certified bereavement facilitator and is board certified in hospice and palliative care nursing. For many years, she was certified in oncology nursing.

From 1980 to 1997, she held the position of oncology clinical specialist at the Veterans Administration Medical Center in Wilkes-Barre, Pennsylvania, and also served as hospice coordinator from the time she initiated the program there in 1982. She has had faculty affiliations at Wilkes University, Penn State University, and two community colleges. She has also presented lectures and research papers at national and international meetings and has published numerous studies, articles, and monographs.

Mrs. Smith is listed in *Who's Who in American Nursing,* has received two awards for excellence in research from the Sigma Theta Tau honor society for nursing, was the 1995 recipient of the Oncology Nursing Society's Quality of Life Lectureship Award, and has served advisory and consultative roles in development of hospice in the Veterans Health Administration. Currently, she is an educational consultant with the Hospice and Palliative Nurses Association and manages a free medical clinic. She resides with her husband, Clair, in Dallas, Pennsylvania.